THE GUT HEALTH SOLUTION

RESTORE DIGESTIVE BALANCE, MANAGE WEIGHT, AND BOOST ENERGY WITH DELICIOUS PROBIOTIC SUPERFOODS

PURE WELLNESS PRESS

Copyright © Pure Wellness Press - All rights reserved.

The content contained within this book may not be reproduced, duplicated or transmitted without direct written permission from the author or the publisher.

Under no circumstances will any blame or legal responsibility be held against the publisher, or author, for any damages, reparation, or monetary loss due to the information contained within this book. Either directly or indirectly. You are responsible for your own choices, actions, and results.

Legal Notice:

This book is copyright protected. This book is only for personal use. You cannot amend, distribute, sell, use, quote or paraphrase any part, or the content within this book, without the consent of the author or publisher.

Disclaimer Notice:

Please note the information contained within this document is for educational and entertainment purposes only. All effort has been executed to present accurate, up to date, and reliable, complete information. No warranties of any kind are declared or implied. Readers acknowledge that the author is not engaging in the rendering of legal, financial, medical or professional advice. The content within this book has been derived from various sources. Please consult a licensed professional before attempting any techniques outlined in this book.

By reading this document, the reader agrees that under no circumstances is the author responsible for any losses, direct or indirect, which are incurred as a result of the use of the information contained within this document, including, but not limited to, — errors, omissions, or inaccuracies.

CONTENTS

Introduction ... 7

1. UNDERSTANDING YOUR GUT MICROBIOME ... 11
   The Gut Microbiome - Your Body's Ecosystem ... 11
   Microbial Diversity and Its Impact on Health ... 12
   The Gut-Brain Axis - Connecting Digestion and Emotion ... 14
   The Role of Environmental Factors in Microbiome Health ... 15

2. DIETARY CHANGES FOR A HEALTHIER GUT ... 19
   Fiber-Rich Foods - Building Blocks of a Healthy Gut ... 19
   Reflection Section ... 21
   Fermented Foods - Nature's Probiotics ... 21
   The Power of Prebiotics - Feeding Your Microbiome ... 23
   Understanding Food Sensitivities - Gluten and Lactose ... 25

3. NATURAL REMEDIES AND HOLISTIC APPROACHES ... 29
   Case Study - A Personal Experience with Essential Oils ... 31
   Fennel and Other Digestive Herbs ... 31
   Mindful Eating - Enhancing Digestion and Satisfaction ... 33

4. LIFESTYLE FACTORS INFLUENCING GUT HEALTH ... 37
   Reflection Section ... 39
   Exercise and Its Effects on the Digestive System ... 39
   The Importance of Sleep in Digestive Health ... 41
   Sustainable Lifestyle Adjustments for Long-Term Health ... 42

5. MANAGING GUT DISORDERS NATURALLY ... 47
   Reflection Section ... 49
   Leaky Gut Syndrome - Understanding and Repairing ... 49
   Reflection Section ... 51

SIBO - Small Intestinal Bacterial Overgrowth
Solutions 51
SIFO - Addressing Intestinal Candida Overgrowth 52
Autoimmune Conditions - Gut Health Connections 54

6. WEIGHT MANAGEMENT AND GUT HEALTH 58
Reflection Section 59
The Role of Probiotics in Weight Regulation 59
The Benefits of an Anti-Inflammatory Diet 60
Blood Type Diets - Personalizing Your Nutrition 62
Carnivore vs. Plant-Based Diets - Pros and Cons 63
Paleo vs. Keto Diets - Pros and Cons 64
Food Combining - Unlocking Digestive Efficiency 65
Intermittent Fasting Techniques - Impact and
Benefits 66

7. ENERGY AND MENTAL CLARITY THROUGH
DIGESTIVE HEALTH 72
Reflection Section 74
Gut Health and Cognitive Function 74
Overcoming Fatigue with Probiotic Superfoods 76
Mental Health Benefits of a Balanced Microbiome 77

8. INTEGRATING INNOVATION AND TECHNOLOGY 80
Reflection Section 81
Online Communities and Support Networks 82
Reflection Section 83
Interactive Quizzes for Personalized Gut Health Plans 83
Utilizing QR Codes for Exclusive Content Access 85

9. COST-EFFECTIVE SOLUTIONS FOR GUT HEALTH 88
Fermentation Checklist 89
Budget-Friendly Superfoods for Digestive Wellness 90
Meal Planning and Preparation on a Budget 92
DIY Remedies for Common Digestive Complaints 94

10. REAL-LIFE SUCCESS STORIES AND TESTIMONIALS 97
Reflection Section 99
Case Studies - Overcoming Chronic Gut Issues 99
Testimonials - The Impact of Lifestyle Changes 101
Lessons Learned - Key Takeaways from Success
Stories 103

11. RECIPES AND MEAL PLANS FOR GUT HEALTH	107
Reflection Section	109
Superfood Smoothies and Infusions	109
Snacks and Desserts - Gut-Friendly Treats	111
Meal Plans for Digestive Wellness	113
12. EMPOWERMENT THROUGH KNOWLEDGE AND SELF-CARE	117
Reflection Section	119
Creating Your Own Gut Health Protocol	119
Long-Term Strategies for Sustained Well-Being	121
13. YOUR DIGESTIVE SYSTEM - AN OVERVIEW	125
Key Digestive Organs	125
Common Digestive Disorders - A Summary	127
Glossary of Terms	131
Conclusion	141
Bibliography	145

"The journey of a thousand miles begins with one step."

— LAO TZU

INTRODUCTION

As I sit here sipping my mug of warm fennel tea, I can't help but reflect on the countless hours I've spent researching, experimenting, and, quite frankly, struggling with my gut health. From the earliest days of my childhood, when lactose intolerance made every ice cream cone a gamble, to the mind-gut challenges that followed me into adulthood, the journey to understanding and nurturing my digestive system has been a long and winding one.

If you're reading this, chances are you've faced your own battles with gut health. Perhaps you've found yourself in the supplement aisle, staring at endless bottles of probiotics and prebiotics, wondering which holds the key to your digestive woes. Or maybe you've spent countless nights tossing and turning, your mind racing as your stomach churns, desperately seeking a solution to the discomfort that plagues you.

You're not alone. Gut health issues have become increasingly prevalent among adults, with millions of people worldwide searching for holistic, integrative approaches to manage their symptoms. From Irritable Bowel Syndrome (IBS) and gluten intolerance to the mind-

INTRODUCTION

gut connection and environmental factors, the complexity of our digestive system can be overwhelming.

That's why I've poured my heart and soul into this book, "The Gut Health Solution: Restore Digestive Balance, Manage Weight, and Boost Energy with Delicious Probiotic Superfoods." Within these pages, you'll find a comprehensive exploration of the key topics surrounding gut health, from the intricacies of the microbiome to the power of fermented foods and natural remedies.

But this isn't just another book on digestive health. It's a deeply personal account of my journey, filled with lessons I've learned through trial and error, diets I've experimented with, and the profound impact that understanding my gut has had on my overall well-being. From the relief I found in the food-combining method to the eye-opening revelations about the role of sugar in fueling "bad" bacteria, I'll share the intimate details of my experiences in the hope they may resonate with your own.

Throughout this book, you'll discover many practical, actionable solutions designed to help you cultivate a healthier digestive system. From easy superfood recipes and budget-conscious meal plans, to sustainable lifestyle adjustments and clear, step-by-step guidance, I've made it my mission to provide you with the tools you need to take control of your gut health.

Now, I want to be clear: I'm not a medical professional. The insights and strategies shared within these pages are based on my experiences and extensive research over the years. While the information provided here can offer relief and support your journey toward better digestive health, you should consult your healthcare provider for advice tailored to your unique needs.

So, what can you expect to gain from this book? By embracing the gut-healthy practices and principles outlined in the following chapters, you may experience improved weight management, increased

INTRODUCTION

energy levels, and enhanced mental clarity. But more than that, you'll embark on a transformative journey of self-discovery, learning to listen to your body's signals and nurture your digestive system with the care and attention it deserves.

I invite you to approach this book with an open mind and a curious spirit. Engage with the content, reflect on your experiences, and, most importantly, be kind to yourself. Remember, this is not a race but a journey where you'll embark on a path toward a happier, healthier, and more vibrant you.

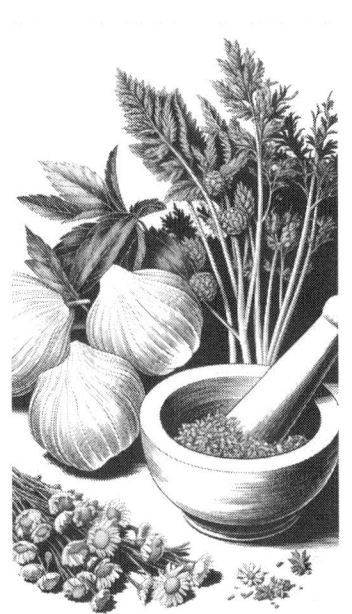

"Every choice you make has an end result."

— ZIG ZIGLAR

1

UNDERSTANDING YOUR GUT MICROBIOME

Have you ever stood in a grocery store aisle, holding a bottle of probiotics, and wondered what these tiny capsules were supposed to do? This chapter is for those who may feel like they're battling a mysterious force within their gut. We'll explore this fascinating internal ecosystem and see why it's crucial to our well-being.

THE GUT MICROBIOME - YOUR BODY'S ECOSYSTEM

Our gut microbiome is like a diverse community where everyone—no matter how small—plays different roles and contributes to the greater good. Scientists have identified thousands of species of friendly bacteria that live in our intestines. These microbes aren't just passive bystanders; they are active participants in our health, working harmoniously to keep everything running smoothly. They interact with each other and with us, their human hosts, creating a symbiotic relationship where both parties benefit.

The microbiome plays a pivotal role in digestion and nutrient absorption, breaking down food particles and making them accessible to our bodies. When you consume a fiber-rich meal, gut bacteria ferment these fibers, producing short-chain fatty acids like butyrate, propionate, and acetate. These fatty acids are more than just byproducts; they provide energy for cells lining the colon and have anti-inflammatory properties.

The microbiome also helps to develop our immune cells, producing antimicrobial proteins and immunoglobulins to defend against harmful pathogens. This intricate relationship with our immune system highlights how interconnected and indispensable these microscopic allies are.

However, when this ecosystem is disturbed, dysbiosis occurs. Dysbiosis is an imbalance within the microbiome, often resulting from antibiotic use, poor diet, or stress. Symptoms like bloating, gas, and irregular bowel movements signal that all is not well. Over time, these imbalances can lead to more significant health issues as the microbiome struggles to perform its essential roles.

Recognizing the signs of dysbiosis allows us to take steps toward restoring balance. Sometimes, we need to take a closer look at what we're feeding our gut microbes—and how external factors like stress may be affecting them. The goal is to nurture this ecosystem, allowing it to sustain us by maintaining the delicate balance essential for optimal health and function.

MICROBIAL DIVERSITY AND ITS IMPACT ON HEALTH

Imagine walking through a vibrant farmer's market. Every stall offers something unique—fruits, vegetables, spices, each contributing to the rich tapestry of aromas and flavors. This diversity is what keeps the market lively and appealing. Your gut microbiome is much like this market; its health and resilience depend on a diverse population of microbes. These microscopic residents form a complex community that works together to fend off diseases, support digestion, and maintain overall health. When we have a wide variety of microbial species, our bodies are better equipped to withstand illnesses and recover swiftly. This diversity reduces the chances of developing inflammatory bowel disease or metabolic syndromes like obesity.

However, several factors can affect the diversity of our gut microbes. Antibiotics and medications, while often necessary in combating harmful bacteria, may also wipe out beneficial microbes, disrupting the balance. This can lead to a decrease in microbial diversity, making the gut more susceptible to imbalances.

Our diets also play a crucial role. A diet rich in processed foods and low in fiber can limit the variety of nutrients available to our gut bacteria, discouraging diversity. On the other hand, a colorful, plant-based diet provides the diverse compounds these microbes thrive on. It is also interesting to note that genetics and early life exposures, like birth delivery methods, can affect our microbiome's initial composition, influencing how it diversifies as we grow.

When diversity diminishes, the consequences can be far-reaching. Reduced microbial variety has been linked to several health conditions. Inflammatory bowel disease is often associated with an imbalanced microbiota, as well as obesity and other metabolic disorders that impact how our bodies process and store nutrients. Even our mental health can be affected. Research links a less diverse gut microbiome to anxiety and depression, highlighting the intricate connections between our gut and brain.

So, how can we strengthen and boost the diversity of our gut's ecosystem? It starts with what we put on our plates. By incorporating a wide range of plant-based foods into our diets, we provide the varied nutrients and fibers that different microbial species need to flourish. Fermented foods and probiotics also offer a rich source of beneficial bacteria that can enhance diversity and support gut health. Foods like yogurt, sauerkraut, and kombucha introduce new microbial strains and enrich the gut environment.

Lifestyle adjustments can also make a significant difference. Reducing stress, getting regular exercise, and prioritizing sleep contribute to a more balanced and diverse microbiome. Each step we take towards nurturing our gut health reflects our overall well-being. The key is to embrace a lifestyle that supports diversity, allowing our gut microbiome to thrive and, in turn, help us through life's many challenges.

THE GUT-BRAIN AXIS - CONNECTING DIGESTION AND EMOTION

Think back to a time when stress weighed heavily on you—perhaps a tight deadline during a hectic workweek or a challenging personal situation. You may have felt your stomach clench or experienced a sudden loss of appetite. This is your gut-brain axis in action, a communication network linking your digestive system and brain. This intricate connection relies on neural pathways and chemical messengers (neurotransmitters) produced by gut bacteria, including serotonin—the 'feel-good' chemical responsible for mood regulation. Remarkably, about 90% of serotonin is produced in the gut, highlighting the microbiome's profound impact on mental well-being.

Research has shown that maintaining a healthy gut can alleviate symptoms of anxiety and depression. Stress can also alter the balance of our microbiome, increasing the production of cortisol, the stress hormone affecting our mental state. Addressing gut health holds the potential to improve mental health. Some studies suggest that gut-targeted therapies, such as probiotics, regulate stress responses and improve mental clarity, offering a holistic approach to managing emotional well-being.

The mechanisms behind this gut-brain connection are fascinating. The vagus nerve, one of the longest nerves in the body, acts as a conduit, transmitting signals between the gut and brain. This nerve also produces neurotransmitters, including serotonin, which modulates mood, sleep, and even appetite. The strength and health of the vagus nerve can significantly impact how these messages are relayed and perceived.

Specific lifestyle changes and dietary adjustments can nurture this intricate connection. Incorporating mind-body practices such as yoga and meditation can enhance the gut-brain axis. These activities promote relaxation, reduce stress, and improve how well the vagus nerve functions. Consuming foods rich in omega-3 fatty acids or antioxidants can support gut and brain health. Foods like fatty fish, nuts, berries, and dark chocolate can be nutritious and delicious ways to lift your mood.

Incorporating these practices into your daily routine can foster a healthier relationship between your gut and brain. Consider setting aside time daily for mindfulness exercises, whether a quick meditation session or a calming yoga practice. Similarly, being mindful of the foods you consume can make a noticeable difference. Try reaching for a handful of walnuts or adding a serving of salmon to your meals to ensure your body receives the nutrients it needs to thrive. These small, consistent efforts can lead to significant improvements in both your digestive and mental health, enhancing your overall quality of life.

THE ROLE OF ENVIRONMENTAL FACTORS IN MICROBIOME HEALTH

It's clear that our environment plays a huge role in shaping our health, particularly when it comes to our gut microbiome. Urban living often brings exposure to pollutants that compromise our microbial balance, impacting how we digest and absorb nutrients.

It's not just the air we breathe but also our choices at home. Looking around your house, you might see various cleaning products and chemicals used to maintain a sparkling clean environment that can disrupt the delicate balance of our gut flora. They can interfere with the microbiome's ability to maintain its diversity and resilience, much like weedkiller, which indiscriminately affects weeds and flowers in a garden.

Then there are medications, particularly antibiotics, which can lead to significant disruptions in our gut microbiome. Antibiotics can eliminate both harmful and beneficial bacteria, leading to a decrease in microbial diversity. This disruption can have long-term consequences, including increased susceptibility to infections and the rise of antibiotic-resistant strains. Over-the-counter (OTC) medications, often relied upon for quick relief from ailments, can also affect the microbiome. Their frequent use can alter gut chemistry, sometimes causing more harm than good. It's important to use medications judiciously and integrate prebiotics and probiotics to help replenish beneficial bacteria to counter these effects.

Diet and nutrition are at the heart of maintaining a healthy microbiome. Processed foods laden with sugar and additives are all convenient, yet can wreak havoc on our gut health. These foods often lack the nutrients necessary to support a diverse and thriving microbiome. Excessive sugar can feed harmful bacteria, tipping the scales toward an imbalance. Alcohol consumption can also impact gut health, altering the microbiome and impairing its function. On the other hand, a diet rich in high-fiber, whole foods can help nurture a robust microbiome. Foods like fruits, vegetables, whole grains, and legumes provide the nutrients and fibers that beneficial bacteria thrive on, encouraging a balanced and healthy gut environment.

We can make several practical changes to protect our microbiome from environmental threats. Choosing organic and natural products reduces exposure to harmful chemicals, supporting a healthier microbiome. Water filtration systems can help remove contaminants from our drinking water, ensuring it doesn't negatively impact our gut flora. Additionally, reducing plastic containers and packaging can prevent harmful chemicals from leaching into our food and beverages, further safeguarding our health.

In reflecting on these aspects of our environment and lifestyle, it becomes clear that while we may not have control over everything, there are steps we can take to protect and nurture our gut health. By making informed choices, whether selecting organic produce or being mindful of medication use, we can create an environment supporting a thriving microbiome. Our gut health doesn't exist in isolation; it's intricately linked to the world around us. By understanding these connections, we empower ourselves to make changes that benefit not just our gut, but our overall well-being. In doing so, we pave the way for a healthier and more vibrant life, one mindful step at a time.

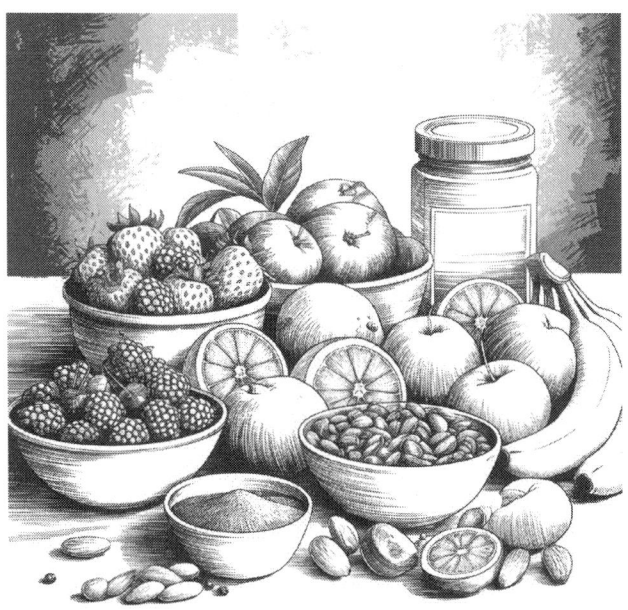

"Let food be thy medicine and medicine be thy food."

— HIPPOCRATES

2

DIETARY CHANGES FOR A HEALTHIER GUT

When I first set out to improve my gut health, I was amazed to learn how essential dietary fiber is to the process. It's the foundation of a healthy digestive system. I remember the moment it clicked—my frequent digestive discomforts weren't random; they were my gut's way of signaling a need for more fiber-rich foods. Yet, modern diets often fall short of the recommended fiber intake, leading to gut issues that many of us mistakenly accept as normal.

FIBER-RICH FOODS - BUILDING BLOCKS OF A HEALTHY GUT

As it turns out, there are different types of fiber playing distinct roles in our digestive system. Soluble fiber is like a sponge, absorbing water and forming a gel-like substance that slows digestion. It isn't a random process; it helps regulate blood sugar levels and keeps cholesterol in check. Insoluble fiber, on the other hand, is the broom of our digestive tract. It adds bulk to stool and helps it pass quickly, preventing constipation. Together, these fibers create a balanced environment in the gut, promoting regularity and preventing many common digestive issues.

Imagine a breakfast of warm oatmeal topped with fresh berries. Oats are an excellent source of soluble fiber, which supports stable energy levels by preventing spikes in blood sugar. For lunch, a hearty quinoa salad can keep you full and satisfied. Quinoa, a whole grain, provides fiber types, supporting your daily digestion. Come dinner, a serving of roasted Brussels sprouts or broccoli offers a fiber-rich side that's both nutritious and delicious. These cruciferous vegetables are packed with insoluble fiber, enhancing bowel regularity and providing a satisfying crunch.

Legumes, like lentils and chickpeas, are another fantastic source of fiber. They not only support gut health but also offer plant-based protein. A lentil soup or a chickpea salad can be a comforting, gentle meal for your digestive system. The beauty of these foods lies in their versatility, allowing you to create diverse and wholesome meals. By incorporating various fiber-rich foods, you can support a healthy gut microbiome essential for overall health.

Understanding the different types of fiber and their functions can help you make informed choices about your diet. While soluble fiber helps slow digestion and regulate blood sugar levels, insoluble fiber is crucial for preventing constipation and maintaining regularity. Both types of fiber are essential for a balanced diet, and consuming a mix of fiber-rich foods can help you meet your daily needs. Aim for a variety of sources, as each food offers unique benefits.

For those new to fiber-rich diets, gradually increasing your intake is essential. A sudden spike in fiber can lead to bloating or discomfort as your gut bacteria adjust to the new influx of nutrients. Start by adding a serving of fiber-rich foods to one meal a day, then slowly incorporate more over time. Drinking plenty of water is also crucial, as it aids in fiber digestion and helps prevent constipation. Staying hydrated ensures fiber can do its job effectively, keeping your digestive system running smoothly.

REFLECTION SECTION

Reflect on your current fiber intake. How often do you include fiber-rich foods in your meals? Consider tracking your meals for a week to identify gaps and opportunities to increase your fiber consumption. Look for simple swaps, like choosing whole grain bread over white or adding a handful of spinach to your morning smoothie. Small changes can significantly impact your gut health, supporting a more balanced and vibrant digestive system.

FERMENTED FOODS - NATURE'S PROBIOTICS

When I first discovered the world of fermented foods, it felt like uncovering a hidden vault of ancient wisdom. These foods, preserved through the ages, enhance our gut health. Fermentation is a natural process where microorganisms like bacteria convert sugars into acids, gases, or alcohol. This transformation extends the shelf life of foods and enriches them with beneficial bacteria that can support our digestive system. Imagine turning a simple cabbage into a probiotic powerhouse, teeming with microbes ready to harmonize with your gut. Fermented foods improve food digestibility, breaking complex carbohydrates into more straightforward, accessible forms. Your body will be able to absorb nutrients more efficiently, reducing the burden on your digestive system and promoting a healthier gut environment.

Fermented foods are not only beneficial but also delightfully diverse. For example, kimchi is a spicy, tangy Korean staple packed with probiotics. Its vibrant flavors come from cabbage, radishes, and spices, all fermented to perfection. Kimchi's rich probiotic content can help balance the gut microbiota, aiding digestion and potentially boosting immunity. Then there's kombucha, a fizzy, refreshing beverage that has recently gained popularity. Kombucha is a probiotic drink that's made from fermented tea and is as enjoyable as it is beneficial. It provides a light, effervescent lift, invigorating the body and the gut. In Japanese cuisine, miso plays a starring role. This savory paste from fermented soybeans is a staple in soups and sauces. Miso is an umami-rich flavor enhancer and a source of probiotics that support a healthy gut.

The magic of fermentation lies in lactic acid bacteria, which play a key role in this transformation. These bacteria thrive in anaerobic conditions, converting sugars into lactic acid. This process not only preserves the food but also enriches it with probiotics. Lactic acid acts as a natural preservative, inhibiting the growth of harmful bacteria and ensuring the longevity of fermented products. It also contributes to the distinct tangy taste characteristic of many fermented foods. This symbiotic relationship between the bacteria and the food creates a nutrient-rich product that can support your digestive system.

Incorporating fermented foods into your diet doesn't have to be daunting. Start with small, manageable changes that fit into your routine. Consider adding a spoonful of sauerkraut to your salads or sandwiches for a tangy twist. Its crunchy texture and probiotic benefits make it a delightful addition to any meal. For a creamy, probiotic-rich breakfast, use yogurt as a base for smoothies. Blend it with your favorite fruits, and you've got a delicious, gut-friendly start to your day. And let's not forget kefir, a cultured dairy drink that's easy to enjoy on its own or mixed with fresh berries. Its mild tang and creamy texture make it a versatile option for those looking to boost their probiotic intake.

Gradually introducing these foods into your diet can help your gut microbiota adjust, minimizing potential digestive discomfort. As you start incorporating more fermented foods, you'll likely notice improved digestion, increased energy, and a more balanced mood. Remember, the goal is to find what works for you, integrating these probiotic-rich foods into your lifestyle in an enjoyable and sustainable way. Your gut will be all the happier for it.

THE POWER OF PREBIOTICS - FEEDING YOUR MICROBIOME

In my quest to nourish my gut, I stumbled upon the understated yet powerful allies known as prebiotics that provide the necessary fuel for probiotics to thrive. For years, eating yogurt every day was enough to keep my body's digestion balanced. But one day, it wasn't. That's when I learned the necessity of prebiotics to feed the probiotics so they'll keep working. Probiotics are the beneficial bacteria that live in our gut, while prebiotics are non-digestible fibers that pass through the digestive system to nourish these bacteria in the colon. Once there, they serve as a feast for the friendly bacteria, promoting their growth and activity. This feast produces short-chain fatty acids (SCFAs), compounds that play a vital role in maintaining gut health and overall well-being.

One of the more intriguing additions to the prebiotic lineup comes from an unexpected source. Turkey Tail, a type of medicinal mushroom, is gaining recognition for its prebiotic properties. Rich in polysaccharides, it supports the gut microbiome by fostering the growth of beneficial bacteria. This mushroom, often found in supplement form, has been a staple in traditional medicine for centuries. Its inclusion in modern prebiotic strategies reflects a harmonious blend of ancient wisdom and contemporary science. By incorporating Turkey Tail into your routine, you may enhance your gut's ability to maintain a balanced microbiome.

In your kitchen, you'll likely find a few prebiotic powerhouses already at your disposal. Garlic and onions, familiar staples in many cuisines, are abundant in inulin—a prebiotic fiber. These aromatic vegetables not only add depth to your dishes but also support the growth of healthy gut bacteria. Asparagus, bananas, cherries and berries are excellent sources of prebiotics. Asparagus is rich in inulin and can be enjoyed steamed or roasted, while bananas offer a convenient snack with the added benefit of prebiotic support. And who doesn't like strawberries or blueberries on their morning cereal? When consumed regularly, these foods can help create a favorable environment for probiotics to flourish.

Understanding the difference between prebiotics and probiotics is crucial for maintaining gut balance. While probiotics are the live bacteria that populate the gut, prebiotics act as their sustenance, ensuring that these beneficial microbes have the energy to colonize and thrive. It's a symbiotic relationship where prebiotics feed the probiotics, enhancing their efficacy and promoting a healthy microbial community. Together, they maintain a harmonious gut environment, supporting digestion and overall health.

Incorporating more prebiotics into your diet doesn't have to be a daunting task. You can start by using chicory root as a coffee substitute. Chicory root is high in inulin and offers a rich, earthy flavor, providing a prebiotic boost with every sip. Leeks, another allium family member, can be added to soups and stews for flavor and prebiotic content. Jerusalem artichokes, often called sunchokes, are another excellent source of inulin. Roasted or sautéed, they can be a delicious addition to your meals. Legumes, grains, and seeds along with tomatoes and avocados are also prebiotics. By being mindful of these choices, you can effortlessly enhance your diet with prebiotics, supporting your gut health in a natural, satisfying way.

It's empowering to know that choosing certain foods can profoundly impact your microbiome and overall sense of vitality. Each meal becomes an opportunity to support your body's intricate systems, allowing you to thrive from the inside out. Whether adding a sprinkle of raw garlic to your salad or sipping on a chicory-infused beverage, these small, intentional steps can significantly improve your digestive health, leaving you feeling more energized and balanced in your daily life.

UNDERSTANDING FOOD SENSITIVITIES - GLUTEN AND LACTOSE

Food sensitivities can feel like an unwelcome guest at a dinner party, making their presence known in the most inconvenient ways. For many, gluten and lactose are the usual suspects, often linked to digestive discomforts that range from mild to downright disruptive. Gluten sensitivity, for instance, can manifest as bloating, diarrhea, or joint pain, leaving individuals feeling off-balance and fatigued. On the other hand, lactose intolerance brings its own suite of symptoms, such as gas, bloating, and cramping, typically occurring within hours of dairy consumption. These reactions are more than just nuisances—they can significantly impact daily life, dictating what and where you can eat.

Lactose intolerance arises from a deficiency in lactase, the enzyme responsible for breaking down lactose, the sugar found in milk and dairy products. Without enough lactase, lactose travels through the gut undigested, leading to fermentation by gut bacteria and the uncomfortable symptoms that follow. Meanwhile, gluten sensitivity or celiac disease involves an immune response to gluten, a protein found in wheat, barley, and rye. This reaction can damage the small intestine's lining, impairing nutrient absorption and causing symptoms beyond digestion.

For those grappling with these sensitivities, finding suitable dietary alternatives is helpful and necessary in maintaining health and enjoyment of food. Gluten-free grains such as rice, millet, and quinoa offer versatile substitutes for various dishes, from breakfast bowls to hearty dinners. For those who miss the creaminess of dairy, lactose-free products and plant-based milks like almond, soy, or oat provide delicious alternatives without the digestive discomfort. Interestingly, some people find relief in consuming milk from brown cows, such as Jerseys or Guernseys, which have a different protein composition than ordinary Holstein milk. Raw milk, though a topic of debate, is also cited by some as a more digestible option due to its natural enzymes.

Identifying food sensitivities can feel like solving a mystery, requiring patience and observation. One effective method is an elimination diet, where you temporarily remove potential trigger foods from your diet, then gradually reintroduce them while monitoring symptoms. This process can help pinpoint specific sensitivities, providing clarity and direction for dietary adjustments. Consulting with healthcare professionals, such as dietitians or allergists, can offer valuable insights and testing options to confirm suspicions and guide dietary planning. Their expertise can help you navigate food sensitivities, ensuring you maintain nutritional balance while avoiding trigger foods.

As you navigate these sensitivities and adapt your diet, remember you're not alone. Many have walked this path and found ways to live fully and joyfully despite dietary restrictions. By understanding your body's unique needs and making informed choices, you can reclaim your relationship with food, turning meals into nourishing, satisfying experiences rather than sources of stress. By embracing dietary changes and exploring new culinary horizons, you'll find a world of delicious, gut-friendly foods ready to bring joy and vitality to your everyday life.

As we wrap up this exploration of dietary changes for a healthier gut, it's clear that what we eat plays a crucial role in our digestive well-being. Each aspect contributes to a balanced gut, from the foundational support of fiber to the probiotic-rich benefits of fermented foods and the nurturing role of prebiotics. Recognizing and addressing food sensitivities further empowers us to tailor our diets to our unique needs, fostering a harmonious relationship with our bodies. This understanding sets the stage for the next chapter, where we'll delve into natural remedies and holistic approaches to support gut health and beyond.

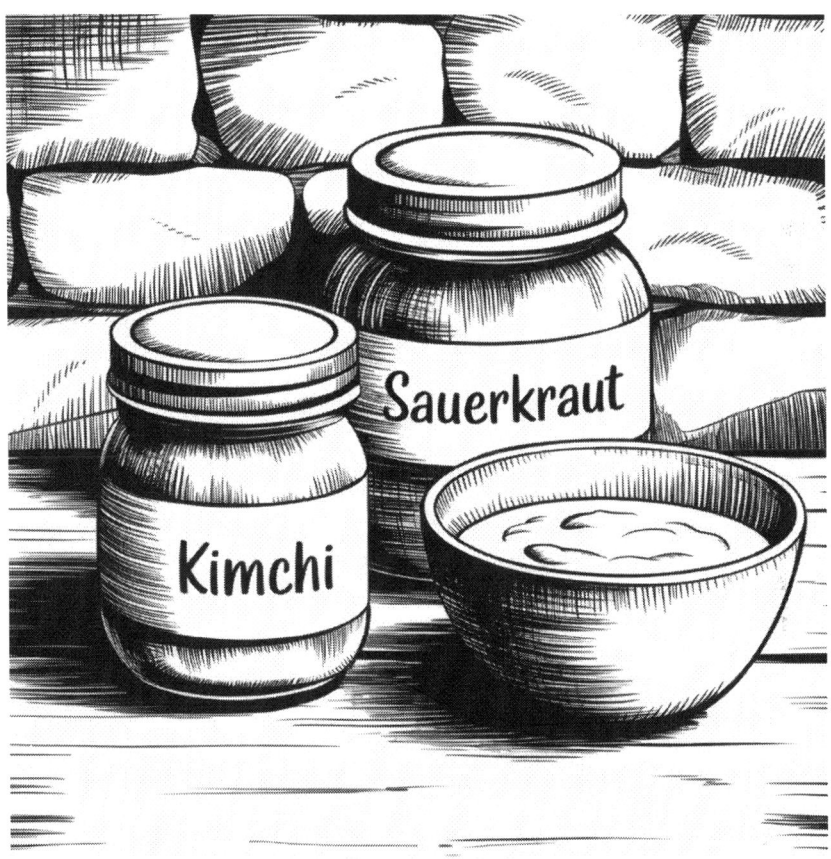

"The journey to wellness starts with a single healthy choice."

— UNKNOWN

3
NATURAL REMEDIES AND HOLISTIC APPROACHES

There's something magical about the world of natural remedies. Just thinking about the vast array of plants and oils, each with its unique properties, every leaf and every petal holding a secret just waiting to be discovered, is something most wonderful. For most of my life, I relied heavily on conventional medicine to address my health concerns, especially when it came to my gut. Yet, the gentle whisper of nature eventually guided me to explore alternative approaches. Essential oils, in particular, captured my attention. Their aromatic allure and potent benefits promised a path to wellness that was both ancient and refreshingly modern.

When discussing food-grade essential oils, we refer to oils safe for culinary use. Food-grade essential oils meet specific criteria for purity and safety. Due to their concentrated nature, they are often used in small quantities to enhance flavor or provide therapeutic benefits. It's essential to approach these oils respectfully and cautiously, recognizing their potency and potential risks.

Peppermint oil, for instance, offers a refreshing flavor and is known for its digestive benefits. Its cooling properties can soothe the symptoms of Irritable Bowel Syndrome (IBS), providing relief from bloating and discomfort. The menthol in peppermint oil relaxes the smooth muscles of the gastrointestinal tract, easing spasms and promoting a sense of calm. In moments of digestive distress, a diluted drop of peppermint oil used safely can offer a gentle reprieve, much like a cool breeze on a sweltering day. Similarly, ginger oil derived from the rhizome of the ginger plant is celebrated for its ability to combat nausea and aid digestion. Its warming, spicy aroma is not only invigorating but also serves as a natural remedy for an upset stomach, making it a staple in many holistic wellness routines.

Safety, however, is paramount when incorporating essential oils into your daily life. The concentration of these oils means that even a single drop carries immense power. Dilution is key. When using essential oils internally, always mix them with a carrier oil, such as coconut or olive oil, to reduce the risk of irritation. A general guideline is to use one drop of essential oil per teaspoon of carrier oil, ensuring a balance that maintains efficacy while prioritizing safety. Some oils, like peppermint and ginger, can also be used in cooking to add flavor and therapeutic benefits. Imagine a warm ginger-infused tea on a chilly morning or a hint of peppermint in a chocolate dessert, both comforting as well as healthful.

While these oils can be a valuable addition to your wellness toolkit, remaining vigilant about their potential risks is crucial. Overuse can lead to adverse effects, from skin irritation to severe digestive issues. Always start with the smallest recommended amount and observe how your body responds. Allergic reactions, such as itching, redness, or swelling, should be taken seriously, and it's wise to discontinue use and consult a healthcare provider if any adverse symptoms arise. The world of essential oils invites curiosity and exploration but demands respect and informed usage.

CASE STUDY - A PERSONAL EXPERIENCE WITH ESSENTIAL OILS

Emily, a dear friend, once shared her experience with me. She had struggled with IBS for years, trying everything from diet changes to prescription medications with little relief. On a whim, Emily decided to try peppermint oil, starting with a single diluted drop in her evening tea. To her surprise, she felt a noticeable reduction in her symptoms. Encouraged by this success, she cautiously introduced ginger oil into her routine, using it in her cooking. Over time, Emily found a balance that worked for her, incorporating these oils into her lifestyle with care and mindfulness. Her story is a testament to the potential of essential oils to support digestive health but also highlights the importance of personalized approaches and awareness.

As we delve into essential oils, remember that their benefits work best when used thoughtfully with other holistic practices. Whether seeking relief from digestive discomfort or exploring new avenues for wellness, essential oils offer a fragrant, fascinating pathway.

FENNEL AND OTHER DIGESTIVE HERBS

In natural remedies, fennel is a time-honored ally for digestive health, its legacy tracing back to ancient civilizations that revered it for its carminative properties. With their gentle, anise-like flavor, these tiny seeds have long been known for their ability to relieve gas and bloating, making them a staple in post-meal rituals across various cultures. The tradition of using fennel as a digestive aid endures today, with fennel tea offering a soothing remedy for those uncomfortable bouts of bloating. Sipping on a warm cup of fennel tea can feel like wrapping your stomach in a comforting embrace, easing tension and promoting a sense of relief. The seeds' high fiber content and anti-inflammatory effects make them a potent tool in maintaining gut harmony.

Yet, fennel is just the beginning. The plant kingdom has a multitude of herbs that cater to our digestive needs, each bringing its unique flair. For example, chamomile's calming properties extend beyond soothing the mind; chamomile is celebrated for relaxing the digestive tract, making it a favorite for those struggling with stomach cramps or indigestion. With its delicate floral notes, a cup of chamomile tea can work wonders on an uneasy stomach, transforming discomfort into tranquility. Then there's licorice root, whose soothing sweetness belies its impressive efficacy against stomach ulcers. This root coats the stomach lining, relieving irritation and supporting natural healing. Its anti-inflammatory compounds help reduce the production of stomach acid, offering a reprieve for those suffering from ulcers. Carom seeds, commonly used in traditional Indian cuisine and Ayurvedic medicine for their effectiveness in treating indigestion, possess antibacterial and anti-inflammatory properties and have also been used to treat peptic ulcers.

Dandelion, often dismissed as a mere weed, is a powerhouse for liver support and detoxification. Its bitter compounds stimulate bile production, aiding digestion and promoting the breakdown of fats. By supporting liver function, dandelion helps cleanse the body of toxins, paving the way for improved digestive health. These herbs' versatility allows for various preparation methods, each unlocking different aspects of their beneficial properties. Herbal infusions and teas are among the most straightforward and effective ways to enjoy their benefits. Simply steeping fennel seeds, chamomile flowers, or dandelion roots in hot water can release their therapeutic compounds, creating a soothing beverage that supports digestion.

Incorporating dried herbs into culinary dishes is another flavorful approach. Imagine adding a sprinkle of fennel seeds to roasted vegetables or incorporating chamomile into baked goods for a sweet, aromatic twist. These small additions can elevate dishes while providing digestive support. The science behind these herbs' efficacy is both fascinating and reassuring. Studies have shown that fennel's carminative properties are due to its volatile oils, which relax intestinal muscles and reduce gas formation. Clinical trials highlight chamomile's anti-inflammatory effects, demonstrating its ability to soothe the digestive tract and relieve symptoms of gastrointestinal distress. These findings confirm what traditional wisdom has long held: that the gifts of nature can play a crucial role in maintaining and restoring digestive health.

MINDFUL EATING - ENHANCING DIGESTION AND SATISFACTION

The benefits of mindful eating extend far beyond the table. By cultivating a more intentional relationship with food, we can alleviate digestive discomfort and enhance nutrient absorption. You might experiment using your non-dominant hand or chopsticks to slow your eating pace, encouraging more deliberate, thoughtful bites. Slowing down allows our bodies to digest food properly, reducing the likelihood of overeating and the bloating that often follows. It gives our brains time to catch up with our stomachs, helping us recognize when we're full. As we become attuned to our hunger and fullness cues, we learn to honor our body's signals, eating when we're hungry and stopping when we're satisfied. This natural rhythm supports healthy digestion and fosters a more balanced relationship with food.

Several exercises can help you develop mindful eating habits. Before eating, try taking a few deep breaths to center yourself. This simple act can calm your mind and prepare you to fully engage with your meal. As you eat, focus on the taste and texture of each bite. Notice how the flavors unfold and how the textures change as you chew. This attention to detail can transform eating into a rich, sensory experience. Keep a mindful eating journal, jotting down your observations about how different foods make you feel physically and emotionally. Reflecting on these insights can deepen your awareness and guide you toward nourishing food choices.

Mindful eating also touches on the psychological and emotional aspects of our relationship with food. By practicing mindfulness, we can reduce the tendency to eat out of stress or boredom, cultivating instead a more positive relationship with food and our bodies. This approach encourages gratitude for the nourishment we receive, fostering a sense of appreciation and respect for the food that sustains us. Over time, mindful eating can help build self-compassion and acceptance, allowing us to let go of guilt or judgment around food choices. Instead, we learn to listen to our bodies with kindness and curiosity, creating a foundation for lasting well-being.

As you explore mindful eating, consider setting aside distractions. Turn off the TV, put away your phone, and focus solely on your meal and the company around you. When we keep mealtimes pleasant, perhaps with light conversation or simply by appreciating the moment, we create an environment that supports both physical and emotional satisfaction. Try setting the table with a nice place setting, even if you are dining alone. Light some candles and use your nice tableware. These small shifts in how we approach meals can significantly change our digestion, satisfaction, and overall health.

Mindful eating is not about strict rules or restrictions. It's about cultivating awareness and presence, allowing each meal to become an opportunity for connection and enjoyment. It's about embracing the journey of nourishment with openness and curiosity, and discovering the joy of eating with intention. As you integrate these practices into your life, you'll likely notice a shift in how you feel physically and emotionally, paving the way for a more harmonious relationship with food and your body.

As we wrap up this exploration of natural remedies and holistic approaches, it's clear that the choices we make each day can have a profound impact on our digestive health. From the calming effects of mindful eating to the powerful support of herbs and oils, these practices invite us to embrace a more intentional, nourishing way of living. As we move forward, we'll continue to uncover the many ways we can support our well-being, exploring the interconnectedness of our body, mind, and spirit.

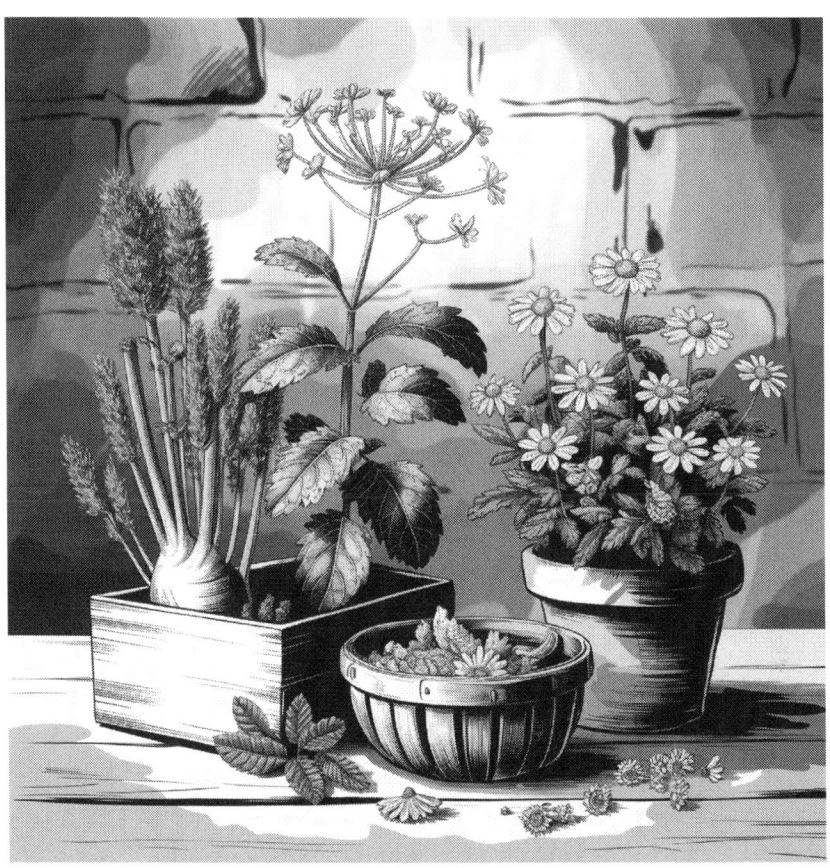

"Tiny changes, remarkable results."

— JAMES CLEAR

4
LIFESTYLE FACTORS INFLUENCING GUT HEALTH

Have you ever noticed how your stomach clenches when you're anxious, or how a wave of nausea seems to hit during a particularly stressful moment? I've experienced this countless times, demonstrating the profound connection between our minds and digestive systems. Stress isn't just a mental state; it can affect our physical being, particularly our gut. This chapter explores how our lifestyle, especially stress, can impact our gut health and what we can do to manage it.

Stress can feel like an unwelcome guest, overstaying its welcome and wreaking havoc on our digestive system. When we're stressed, our body activates the gut-brain axis, a communication network between the brain and the gut. This activation can alter gut motility, meaning the movement of food and waste through the digestive tract, which leads to symptoms like bloating, diarrhea, or constipation. Chronic stress can even impair the microbiota-gut-brain axis, disrupting the communication between our gut and brain. Over time, the burden of stress can accumulate, potentially contributing to disorders like Irritable Bowel Syndrome (IBS) and even affecting mental health. Understanding this relationship is crucial for managing stress and supporting our gut health.

Managing stress is not just about finding moments of relaxation; it's about creating a toolkit of techniques to help reduce its impact on digestion. Mindfulness meditation is a powerful practice that encourages us to focus on the present moment, fostering a sense of calm and reducing the stress response. By spending just a few minutes each day in meditation, you can begin to quiet the mind and soothe the gut. Breathing exercises, such as deep diaphragmatic breathing, can also be incredibly effective. Taking slow, deep breaths activates the parasympathetic nervous system, which helps counteract the stress response and promotes relaxation.

Progressive muscle relaxation, where you tense and slowly release each muscle group, can further ease tension and encourage a state of calm. Yoga is an excellent practice where mindfulness and focus is practiced for stress release.

The benefits of reducing stress for digestion are significant. By managing stress, you can decrease symptoms of IBS, resulting in a more comfortable and regular digestion. Stress reduction also enhances nutrient absorption, ensuring that your body can effectively utilize the nutrients from the food you eat. Not only does your gut feel better, your overall health improves as well. Digestion becomes more efficient, and the uncomfortable symptoms associated with stress-induced gut issues diminish.

Incorporating stress management techniques into daily life may seem challenging, especially with a busy schedule. However, there are practical ways to make it work. Set aside a few minutes each day for relaxation activities, whether it's meditation, a short walk, or simply sitting quietly. Digital tools and apps, like *Calm* or *Headspace*, offer guided sessions that can fit into any routine, making stress reduction accessible and convenient. These tools can be a great starting point for building a consistent stress management practice. Remember, even small steps can make a difference; the key is consistency. By integrating these practices into your life, you support not only your gut health but your overall well-being.

REFLECTION SECTION

Think about a recent stressful event and how it affected your digestion. How did your body react? Write down your observations, then consider which stress management technique might help you the next time a similar situation arises. Try practicing this technique regularly, even when you're not stressed, to build resilience and support your gut health.

EXERCISE AND ITS EFFECTS ON THE DIGESTIVE SYSTEM

One of the biggest surprises in my exploration of gut health was the impact of physical activity on our digestive system. As someone who has always struggled to find motivation for regular exercise, discovering its benefits for gut health was a game changer.

Regular movement is like a gentle massage for the intestines, promoting regular bowel movements and preventing constipation. By increasing blood flow and oxygen delivery to the gut, exercise encourages the production of digestive enzymes, which are crucial for breaking down food and absorbing nutrients. This process enhances digestive wellness and contributes to overall health, boosting energy levels and vitality.

Many options are available when choosing the right type of exercise for digestive health. Low-impact activities like walking and yoga are incredibly beneficial. A brisk walk can stimulate the digestive tract, helping to move food along more efficiently. Yoga, with its various poses and focus on deep breathing, enhances circulation and relaxes the digestive muscles, relieving bloating and discomfort. High-intensity interval training (HIIT) is an excellent choice for those who enjoy more intensity. This exercise boosts metabolism, which can encourage a healthy balance of gut bacteria and improve gut motility, or the movement of the digestive tract. The key is finding activities you enjoy, making it easier to maintain a consistent routine.

The science behind these benefits speaks to the interconnectedness of our body's systems. Exercise promotes an increase in gut microbial diversity, which is vital for a resilient and healthy microbiome. A diverse microbiome can better protect against pathogens, support immune function, and enhance nutrient absorption. Physical activity also encourages the release of endorphins, our body's natural feel-good chemicals, which can reduce stress and improve gut health indirectly. By enhancing gut motility, exercise helps maintain a regular rhythm in our digestive tract, reducing the chances of constipation and other digestive issues.

Incorporating exercise into daily life doesn't have to be overwhelming. Start by creating a workout schedule that fits your lifestyle. If you're new to exercise, begin with short walks around your neighborhood or gentle yoga sessions at home. As you build stamina, gradually increase the intensity and duration of your workouts. Incorporate movement into your daily activities by taking the stairs instead of the elevator, parking further from the store, or even dancing to your favorite music at home. These small choices add up and can significantly benefit your gut health. Aim for at least 30 minutes of moderate physical activity, and remember that consistency is key. The goal is to find a routine that suits your interests and schedule, making it an enjoyable part of your day.

It's important to listen to your body and choose activities that feel good. Consider consulting a healthcare professional before starting a new exercise regimen if you have any medical conditions or concerns. They can provide personalized guidance and ensure your chosen activities are safe and appropriate for your needs. Remember that the best exercise is the one you'll do regularly, so focus on finding activities that bring you joy and fulfillment. By prioritizing movement, you'll support your digestive health, improve your overall quality of life, and feel more energized.

THE IMPORTANCE OF SLEEP IN DIGESTIVE HEALTH

Sleep regulates many bodily functions, including digestion. When we don't get enough rest, our gut integrity can suffer. Studies have shown that sleep deprivation can negatively affect the gut lining, making it more permeable and susceptible to inflammation. Inadequate sleep can disrupt the production of hormones crucial for regulating appetite, such as ghrelin and leptin, which can lead to overeating or poor food choices.

Inadequate sleep can create a ripple effect on digestion, increasing the risk of gastrointestinal disorders. Conditions like IBS can become exacerbated when our sleep patterns are irregular or insufficient. Like our sleep-wake cycle, our digestive system follows a natural circadian rhythm. When sleep is disrupted, so too is this digestive rhythm, leading to issues such as indigestion or irregular bowel movements. Additionally, the lack of restorative sleep can impair the body's ability to repair and rejuvenate, leaving us more vulnerable to digestive disturbances and other health issues.

Improving sleep quality can be transformative for gut health, and there are several strategies to help achieve better rest. Establishing a consistent sleep schedule is an important first step. Going to bed and waking up at the same time each day helps to regulate your body's internal clock, making it easier to fall asleep and wake up naturally. Creating a restful sleep environment can also make a significant difference. Consider making your bedroom a sanctuary by reducing noise, keeping the room cool, and using blackout curtains. Eating meals well ahead of bedtime is another practical strategy. It gives your body time to digest food before lying down, reducing the risk of discomfort or acid reflux. Limiting screen time before bed can also enhance sleep quality, as the blue light emitted by phones and computers can interfere with the production of melatonin, the hormone that regulates sleep.

The relationship between sleep and gut health is bidirectional, meaning a healthy gut can also promote better sleep. Our gut bacteria play a role in producing neurotransmitters that affect sleep, like serotonin, which is a precursor to melatonin. A balanced gut microbiome can support the production of these chemicals, enhancing sleep quality. Some gut bacteria can influence sleep patterns, demonstrating the interconnectedness of our body's systems. By nurturing your gut health, you may find that your sleep improves, which benefits your overall well-being.

Recognizing this connection, I've consciously prioritized my sleep, knowing it supports my digestive health and that each part of our lifestyle plays a role in how we feel. As I've found, and I hope you will too, investing in better sleep is one of the most worthwhile gifts we can give ourselves, paving the way for a healthier, more balanced life.

SUSTAINABLE LIFESTYLE ADJUSTMENTS FOR LONG-TERM HEALTH

When I started looking into improving my gut health, I was inundated with quick fixes and fad diets that promised miraculous results. But deep down, I knew that real, lasting change required sustainable adjustments—small, manageable shifts that could seamlessly fit into my everyday life. The key was gradually building habits, like planting and nurturing seeds in a garden to have a beautiful bloom and yield. This approach is more practical and forgiving, allowing us time to adapt and grow without the pressure of perfection.

One of the first areas I focused on was my diet, prioritizing whole, unprocessed foods. By choosing foods in their natural state, I consumed more nutrients and fewer additives. This shift wasn't about restriction but rather about embracing various colorful fruits and vegetables, lean proteins, and healthy fats. Whole foods support a balanced gut microbiome, providing the fibers and compounds that beneficial bacteria thrive on. Over time, this change became less of a conscious effort and more of a natural preference as my body began to crave the nourishment these foods provided. I also became more mindful of my sugar intake, starting with cutting out soda due to its high sugar content. I replaced it with water infused with berries or cucumber slices for a refreshing alternative. Over time, I realized I didn't miss cola at all. When I finally tried it again after several years, I was surprised to find that I no longer enjoyed the taste.

Another significant adjustment was reducing exposure to environmental toxins. I started by examining the products I used daily, from cleaning supplies to personal care items. Another simple yet effective change was choosing eco-friendly household products. By selecting items made from natural ingredients and sustainable materials, I minimized my exposure to harmful chemicals while supporting environmentally conscious practices. This adjustment aligned with my values, creating a harmonious living environment supporting my health and the planet. Switching to eco-friendly alternatives supported my gut health and felt like a step toward a more sustainable lifestyle. It was a reminder that our environment plays a crucial role in our well-being, and small changes can have a significant impact. Opting for natural products free from harsh chemicals allowed me to create a safer space for myself and my family.

Beyond physical health, enhancing social connections was a vital and necessary component of my well-being. Engaging with others and fostering meaningful relationships contributed to mental wellness, which in turn supported my physical health. Whether joining a community group, attending local events, or simply spending more quality time with loved ones, these interactions helped reduce stress and provided a sense of belonging. Engaging in community activities became a source of fulfillment and stress relief. Whether volunteering, joining a local club, or participating in neighborhood events, these activities enriched my life and provided opportunities to connect with like-minded individuals. The sense of community and shared purpose helped to ground me, offering support and encouragement in my health journey. The emotional support and shared experiences strengthened my resilience, making it easier to maintain healthy habits.

Meal prepping became a practical strategy to avoid processed foods and ensure I had healthy options readily available. By dedicating a few hours each week to planning and preparing meals, I could resist the temptation of convenience foods, knowing I had nourishing meals waiting for me at home. This supported my gut health, saved time, and reduced stress during busy days. It was a small investment with significant returns, helping me to stay on track with my dietary goals.

The process of habit formation played a crucial role in achieving these sustainable changes. Consistency and routine became my allies, guiding me through the ups and downs of lifestyle adjustments. Using habit-tracking tools helped me maintain focus, offering a visual reminder of my progress and areas for improvement. Whether it was a simple checklist or dedicated app, these tools kept me accountable and motivated, reinforcing the positive changes I was making.

As we close this chapter, it's clear that sustainable lifestyle adjustments are key to long-term health. By prioritizing whole foods, reducing toxins, and nurturing social connections, we lay the groundwork for a balanced, supportive environment that fosters well-being. The journey may be gradual, but each step brings us closer to a healthier, more vibrant life. In the next chapter, we'll explore how dietary changes can further enhance gut health, building on the foundation we've established here.

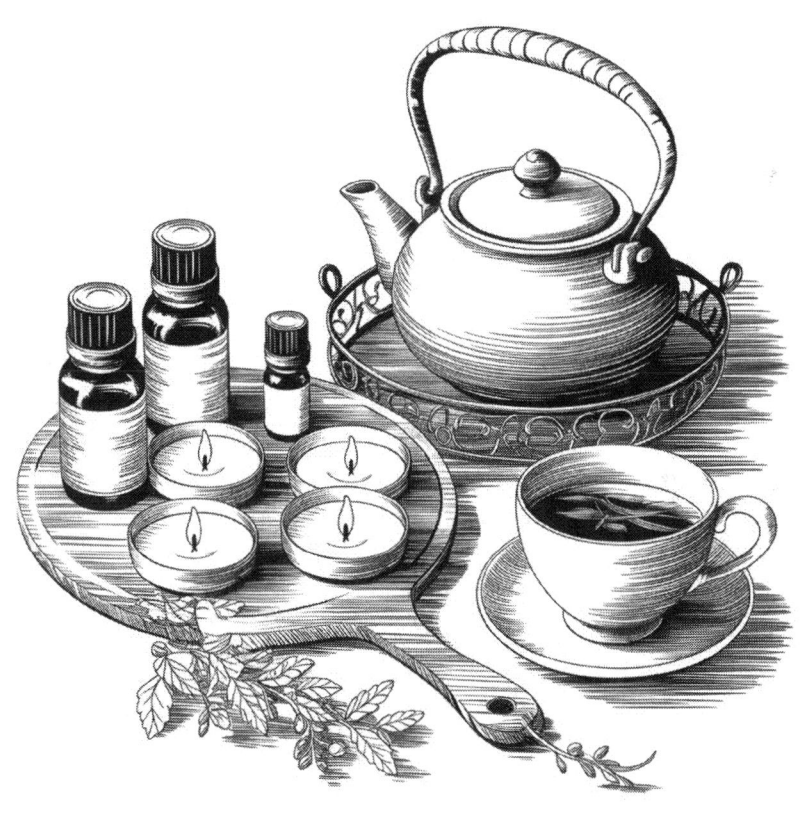

"Be patient and trust the process."

— UNKNOWN

5
MANAGING GUT DISORDERS NATURALLY

I remember sitting at my kitchen table one morning, sipping a cup of herbal tea, feeling the familiar twinges of discomfort in my belly. It was a routine I knew all too well, the ebb and flow of digestive unrest that seemed to have its own agenda. Like many, I was navigating the world of Irritable Bowel Syndrome (IBS), a condition that's a game of trial and error, where the rules change without notice, and understanding the triggers is half the battle. IBS can be quite the chameleon, with symptoms influenced by various factors, leaving many of us feeling bewildered.

One of the primary culprits is diet. Certain food groups can trigger IBS symptoms, turning a pleasant meal into a cause for concern. High-fat foods, dairy, fruits, and vegetables can induce bloating and discomfort. The complexity of IBS makes it crucial to identify personal food triggers. Psychological stress also plays a significant role. Stress doesn't only affect the mind; it echoes in the gut, magnifying symptoms and leaving us anxious about the next flare-up. Hormonal changes can cause IBS flare-ups as well, with fluctuations intensifying symptoms.

Navigating the dietary maze of IBS can feel daunting, but adopting a low-FODMAP diet can help. This approach focuses on reducing fermentable oligosaccharides, disaccharides, monosaccharides, and polyols—complex carbohydrates that can be tough on the gut for a short time. By limiting these, you can alleviate symptoms and find some digestive peace. Gradual reintroduction of potentially triggering foods helps pinpoint specific sensitivities, allowing for a more personalized diet. It's a process that requires patience and careful observation, but the relief it brings is worth the effort. Another option is to permanently eliminate the consumption of all complex carbohydrates to reduce these unpleasant symptoms. The Specific Carbohydrate Diet (SCD) diet that deals with this is not easy, but may bring much-needed relief.

Stress management is equally vital in the battle against IBS. Cognitive behavioral therapy (CBT) can be a powerful ally, helping you change negative thought patterns and thus reduce stress. By addressing the emotional aspects, you can lessen the physical symptoms. Relaxation exercises tailored for IBS sufferers, such as deep breathing or progressive muscle relaxation, offer tangible ways to calm the nervous system and the gut. These practices, integrated into daily life, can be transformative, providing tools to navigate stress in a better and more healthy way.

There are promising options for those seeking alternative therapies. Peppermint oil capsules can help reduce spasms, offering relief from cramps and discomfort. Acupuncture, an ancient practice, has shown promise in managing IBS symptoms, helping to balance the body's energies, and promoting healing. Some studies suggest that acupuncture may help reduce gut inflammation, improve digestion, and relieve symptoms by promoting relaxation, improving blood flow, and regulating the nervous system. These natural remedies create a holistic approach to managing IBS when used alongside dietary and lifestyle changes. They offer a path to relief that respects the body's rhythms and needs.

Reiki, another alternative practice, may support gut health by helping reduce stress and tension, common contributors to digestive issues, while promoting relaxation and enhancing energy flow throughout the body. This can potentially ease discomfort associated with conditions like indigestion or IBS. In traditional Eastern medicine and energy healing, the solar plexus chakra—situated above the navel—is linked to digestion, nutrient absorption, and the wellbeing of the stomach, liver, and gallbladder. Reiki practitioners often work to balance and clear this energy center to encourage digestive harmony. While there are anecdotal reports of Reiki benefiting gut health, scientific research on its direct effects remains limited. It should be viewed as a complementary practice rather than a substitute for conventional medical treatment.

REFLECTION SECTION

Consider keeping a food and symptom journal to identify your IBS triggers. Document what you eat, note any symptoms, and reflect on potential patterns. This practice can provide valuable insights, empowering you to make informed choices and regain control over your digestive health.

LEAKY GUT SYNDROME - UNDERSTANDING AND REPAIRING

Leaky gut syndrome sounds almost fictional but is gaining attention for its potential impact on overall health. Imagine your intestinal lining as a vigilant gatekeeper, controlling what enters your bloodstream. It's a single-cell-thick barrier, allowing nutrients to pass through while keeping harmful substances out. But sometimes, this barrier is compromised, and increased intestinal permeability occurs. This is what we refer to as a "leaky gut." When this happens, larger molecules slip through, potentially igniting inflammation and disrupting immune function. Factors like poor diet, chronic stress, or long-term medication can all contribute to this increased permeability, challenging the gut's integrity.

Recognizing leaky gut isn't always straightforward, as symptoms can mimic other conditions. Chronic fatigue, joint pain, and digestive discomfort are common indicators, but they often go unnoticed or misattributed. Some people experience food sensitivities, skin issues, or even mood changes. Diagnosing leaky gut can involve tests such as lactulose-mannitol, which measures how well your gut absorbs these two sugars. While it sounds technical, this test offers insight into your gut's permeability. If you suspect a leaky gut, guidance from a healthcare provider who understands gut health can be invaluable.

Addressing a leaky gut starts with nourishing the intestinal lining. Dietary strategies play a vital role in this repair process. Bone broth, rich in collagen, supports the gut lining's integrity. It's like giving your gut a warm hug, providing the building blocks it needs to heal. L-glutamine, an amino acid, is another powerful ally known for its ability to repair and maintain the gut barrier. This supplement can easily be incorporated into your routine, offering targeted support. Probiotic-rich foods, such as yogurt or kefir, help restore balance, promoting a healthy microbiome that can protect against further permeability.

Lifestyle changes are equally important in supporting gut healing. Reducing exposure to environmental toxins, like those found in processed foods or certain household products, can lighten the load on your gut. Consider swapping out chemical-laden cleaners for natural alternatives, or choosing organic produce to minimize pesticide intake. Incorporating anti-inflammatory practices into your daily routine can also aid in gut repair. Mindful eating, regular physical activity, and stress-reduction techniques benefit the gut and enhance overall wellness. They encourage the body to shift from a state of chronic stress to one of healing and balance.

REFLECTION SECTION

Take a moment to consider your daily habits. Are there areas where you might reduce exposure to toxins or incorporate more anti-inflammatory practices? Start with a tiny change, like switching to organic produce or trying a new relaxation technique. Reflect on how these adjustments make you feel, and keep a journal to track any changes in symptoms or overall well-being. Your gut—and your whole body—will thank you for it.

SIBO - SMALL INTESTINAL BACTERIAL OVERGROWTH SOLUTIONS

I remember the day I first heard about SIBO—Small Intestinal Bacterial Overgrowth. It was like a light bulb went off, illuminating the possible cause behind the constant bloating and digestive discomfort I had been battling. SIBO occurs when bacteria, typically found in other parts of the gut, colonize the small intestine. This bacterial overgrowth can lead to symptoms like bloating, gas, and nutrient deficiencies. Unlike other gut disorders, SIBO is unique because it involves bacteria thriving where they shouldn't, disrupting normal digestive processes. The excess bacteria can interfere with nutrient absorption, leading to deficiencies in vital vitamins and minerals, such as vitamin B12. Recognizing these signs is crucial because they can easily be mistaken for other conditions, leaving many of us suffering in silence.

Understanding what causes SIBO can be a game-changer in managing it. Reduced motility, or the slowed movement of food through the digestive tract, is a major contributor. When food lingers too long, it provides a feast for bacteria, allowing them to multiply unchecked. Previous antibiotic use also plays a role. While antibiotics are effective at treating infections, they can disrupt the balance of gut bacteria, setting the stage for overgrowth when conditions allow. A complex interplay of factors can tip the scales toward SIBO, making it a challenging condition to tackle.

Addressing SIBO naturally involves a blend of dietary and herbal interventions. The Specific Carbohydrate Diet (SCD) offers a structured approach by eliminating complex carbohydrates that feed bacterial overgrowth. This diet focuses on simple, easily digestible foods, reducing the fuel available to harmful bacteria. Herbal antimicrobials like berberine can also be effective. Berberine's antibacterial properties can help control overgrowth, offering a more natural alternative to antibiotics. Coupling these with a low-FODMAP diet can alleviate symptoms by removing foods that ferment in the gut, minimizing discomfort and bloating.

Preventing SIBO from returning requires vigilance and proactive management. Regular monitoring of symptoms and dietary adjustments help keep bacteria in check. It's like tending a garden; consistent care prevents weeds from taking over. Gut motility exercises, such as yoga or gentle abdominal massage, can support the natural movement of the digestive tract, reducing the risk of stagnation. These exercises encourage the rhythmic contractions that propel food through the intestines, keeping everything moving as it should. By nurturing your digestive system with mindful practices and supportive dietary choices, you lay the foundation for a healthier gut.

SIFO - ADDRESSING INTESTINAL CANDIDA OVERGROWTH

Intestinal Candida Overgrowth, often called SIFO—Small Intestinal Fungal Overgrowth, might sound like something from a science fiction novel, but it's a condition many people grapple with. It's essentially an overgrowth of the yeast candida in the small intestine. While candida is a fungus that naturally resides in our bodies, it can become problematic when it grows beyond normal bounds. This overgrowth can lead to frustratingly familiar symptoms, often challenging to pinpoint, such as persistent bloating and fatigue. Unlike bacterial overgrowth like SIBO, which involve bacteria flourishing in the wrong part of the gut, SIFO is about yeast taking center stage. Understanding this distinction is crucial for anyone looking to manage their symptoms effectively.

Addressing SIFO requires a thoughtful approach, beginning with dietary changes that target yeast balance. The anti-candida diet focuses on reducing sugar intake, as sugar is a favorite fuel source for candida. By cutting back on sugars and refined carbs, you can help starve the overgrowth, making it less likely to thrive. This means saying goodbye to sugary desserts and processed snacks, but it doesn't have to be a flavorless journey. Incorporating whole foods, rich in nutrients but low in sugars, can make the transition manageable and enjoyable. Lean proteins, fresh vegetables, and healthy fats become your allies in restoring balance. Additionally, lifestyle changes such as reducing stress and getting enough sleep can support your body's efforts to combat overgrowth, as a well-rested, less-stressed body is more resilient against infections.

Probiotics and antifungal herbs can be pivotal in managing intestinal candida overgrowth. Saccharomyces boulardii, a beneficial yeast, has been shown to help balance yeast levels in the gut. It works by competing with candida for resources, effectively keeping its numbers in check. Introducing S. boulardii into your routine, whether through supplements or fermented foods, can support your gut in maintaining equilibrium. On the herbal front, oregano oil emerges as a natural antifungal agent. The potent properties of oregano oil can help reduce candida levels and relieve symptoms. However, it's crucial to use it wisely, as its strong nature requires careful dosing.

Prevention and management of SIFO involve a combination of dietary vigilance and regular monitoring. Implementing a low-

FODMAP diet can reduce symptoms by minimizing the foods that ferment in your gut, which candida loves. Keeping a food diary can help you stay on track, allowing you to identify any food-related triggers. It's also wise to consult a healthcare provider familiar with gut health, who can offer personalized advice and track your progress. Regular check-ins can ensure that you're managing symptoms and addressing any underlying issues that may contribute to overgrowth. By taking these steps, you can work toward a healthier gut environment that is less hospitable to candida and more supportive of your overall well-being.

AUTOIMMUNE CONDITIONS - GUT HEALTH CONNECTIONS

I've often marveled at how interconnected our bodies are, especially regarding the gut and immune system. It's like a finely tuned orchestra, where each section plays its part to create harmony. Unfortunately, with autoimmune diseases, something goes awry, and our immune system, designed to protect us, mistakenly attacks our own tissues. Gut permeability, the so-called "leaky gut," actually influences the development of autoimmune conditions. When the intestinal barrier is compromised, larger particles slip through, triggering an immune response. This leads to inflammation, setting the stage for autoimmune disorders.

The gut microbiota, the trillions of microbes in our digestive tract, also influence immune function. They communicate with immune cells, helping maintain balance and preventing unnecessary attacks on the body's tissues. When this balance is disrupted, it can exacerbate autoimmune conditions. Specific diseases, like celiac disease and Hashimoto's thyroiditis, highlight this connection. Celiac disease is characterized by an immune response to gluten, leading to damage in the small intestine. Hashimoto's thyroiditis, an autoimmune condition affecting the thyroid, is another example where gut health considerations come into play. Research suggests that gut dysbiosis may contribute to the development and progression of this disease.

Diet and lifestyle choices can profoundly impact our gut health and, by extension, autoimmune conditions. The Autoimmune Protocol (AIP) diet is one approach that seeks to reduce inflammation and support the gut. It removes potential irritants, like grains and dairy, while emphasizing nutrient-dense foods such as vegetables, fruits, and quality proteins. The goal is to provide the body with anti-inflammatory nutrients to help modulate the immune response. Incorporating anti-inflammatory practices, like regular exercise and stress reduction techniques, can further support this process. These lifestyle changes can help create an environment where the body can heal and thrive.

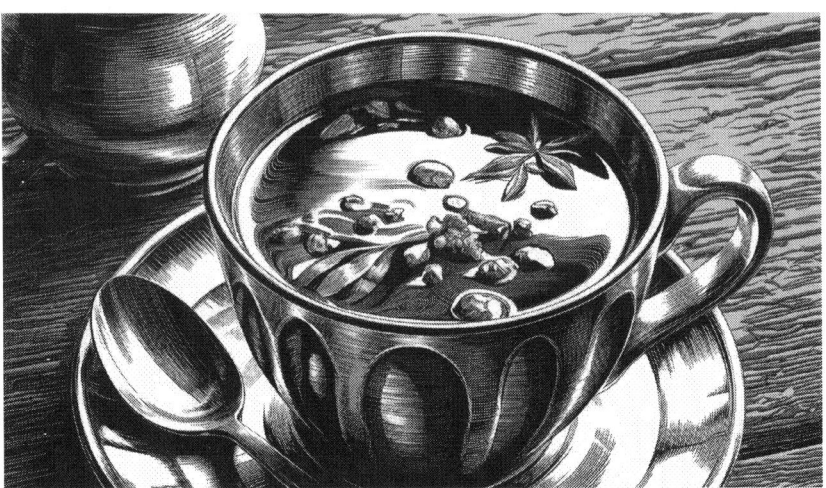

Probiotics and prebiotics also play a role in managing autoimmune conditions. Certain probiotic strains, like Lactobacillus and Bifidobacterium, have been shown to support gut health and modulate immune responses. They can help maintain a balanced microbiota, which prevents dysregulation. Prebiotic foods, like garlic, onions, and asparagus, enhance gut microbiota diversity by feeding beneficial bacteria. This diversity is key to a resilient immune system, capable of differentiating between friend and foe. Incorporating these elements into your diet can support your gut health and potentially influence autoimmune conditions.

As we finish this chapter, it's clear that our gut health is key to understanding and managing many autoimmune conditions. The path forward involves a holistic approach, considering diet, lifestyle, and the profound connection between our gut and immune system. These insights offer hope for those seeking relief and a more balanced life. As we explore the intricacies of gut health, we'll uncover more ways to nurture our bodies and promote well-being.

"The more you know, the better choices you make."

— OPRAH WINFREY

6

WEIGHT MANAGEMENT AND GUT HEALTH

Remember when you realized your favorite pair of jeans felt just a tad too tight? It was a wake-up call for me, too. I wondered if my gut health had anything to do with it. Surprisingly, our gut flora plays a pivotal role in how our bodies manage weight. The gut is home to trillions of bacteria, and these microbes are not just passive passengers. They actively break down complex carbohydrates that our bodies can't digest on their own. By fermenting these carbohydrates, gut bacteria produce short-chain fatty acids that provide energy and regulate fat storage. This bacterial activity influences whether those jeans fit comfortably or not.

Our gut bacteria also help regulate energy expenditure, impacting metabolic processes in subtle yet significant ways. They interact with hormones like insulin, which controls blood sugar levels and affects how efficiently our bodies burn calories. A diverse gut microbiome is crucial for maintaining insulin sensitivity and ensuring glucose is metabolized effectively. When the microbiome is out of balance, it can lead to metabolic disorders, contributing to weight gain and conditions like obesity. Dysbiosis, a term for microbial imbalance, can trigger inflammation, leading to insulin resistance and potentially type 2 diabetes.

Optimizing gut flora is key to supporting metabolic health and can be achieved through dietary changes. Incorporating a variety of plant-based foods not only feeds the beneficial bacteria but also promotes microbial diversity. Think of your gut as a garden; the more diverse the plants, the healthier the ecosystem. Regular consumption of fermented foods like kimchi, sauerkraut, and yogurt introduce new strains of beneficial bacteria, enhancing gut health. These foods support digestion and also contribute to a balanced metabolism, which in turn supports our weight management goals.

REFLECTION SECTION

Consider keeping a weekly food diary to track your diet and its effects on your gut health. Note any changes in digestion or energy levels when you include more plant-based and fermented foods. Reflect on these observations to understand how your dietary choices influence your weight management journey.

THE ROLE OF PROBIOTICS IN WEIGHT REGULATION

I remember the first time I heard about probiotics and their potential impact on weight. It seemed far-fetched, but the more I learned, the more it made sense. Specific strains of probiotics, like Lactobacillus gasseri, have been shown to influence abdominal fat. This strain can target the stubborn fat that often clings to our midsections, a problem many of us are familiar with. Bifidobacterium lactis is another probiotic that plays a role in weight control, helping to maintain a balance in our gut microbiota that supports a healthy body composition.

Probiotics work their magic by altering the gut microbiota composition, affecting weight regulation. They can modulate appetite-regulating hormones like ghrelin and peptide YY, which signal hunger and satiety to your brain. This means you may feel full sooner, helping to curb overeating. Probiotics also help enhance gut barrier function, reducing inflammation that can lead to weight gain. A healthy gut barrier functions like a fortified castle, blocking harmful invaders while safeguarding your body's optimal performance.

Choosing the right probiotic supplement for weight management involves more than just grabbing the first bottle you see. It's crucial to consider strain-specific research, as not all probiotics have the same effects. Look for strains like Lactobacillus gasseri or Bifidobacterium lactis, which have shown promising results in studies. The dosage and delivery method matter, too. Some probiotics are more effective when taken in specific forms, like capsules or powders, which can ensure they reach your gut alive. It pays to do some homework and consult a healthcare professional to find a probiotic that suits your needs.

Prebiotics, the non-digestible fibers that feed probiotics, can enhance probiotic effects. They create a symbiotic relationship that boosts gut health and supports weight management. Foods rich in prebiotics, such as garlic, onions, and bananas, can be easily incorporated into your diet to complement probiotic supplements. The mushroom mycelium, Turkey Tail, is a natural prebiotic supplement that supports probiotics in your microbiome and makes them more effective. This synergy can make a noticeable difference in how your body processes and stores fat, ultimately influencing your weight management efforts.

THE BENEFITS OF AN ANTI-INFLAMMATORY DIET

An anti-inflammatory diet might sound trendy, but it's grounded in reducing inflammation throughout the body, including the gut. The Autoimmune Protocol or AIP diet emphasizes whole, unprocessed foods—the kind our ancestors would have recognized. Whole foods like fruits, vegetables, and grains provide the nutrients and antioxidants needed to combat inflammation and support gut health. Think of it as giving your body a toolkit to repair and maintain itself.

Selecting the right foods is key to making a significant impact. Omega-3 fatty acid-rich fatty fish such as salmon and mackerel exhibit strong anti-inflammatory effects. Similarly, leafy greens such as spinach and kale are abundant in vitamins and minerals, aiding in calming the body's inflammatory responses. On the flip side, it's beneficial to avoid trans fats and processed sugars, notorious for intensifying inflammation and disturbing gut health, and commonly found in processed snacks and fast foods. The diet initially recommends avoiding certain foods and beverages known to potentially exacerbate inflammation. This includes coffee and alcohol, along with a group of vegetables known as nightshades, which encompass eggplant, tomatoes, peppers, and potatoes. Additionally, it suggests temporarily eliminating grains, nuts, seeds, and dairy products from your diet. These items are reintroduced later, one at a time, to monitor for potential adverse reactions. By adopting these mindful dietary alterations, you can tailor a diet that fortifies your body's natural healing mechanisms.

Reducing inflammation extends beyond gut health. It alleviates digestive disorders, providing relief from conditions like IBS or Crohn's disease. Aloe vera juice is a natural remedy for soothing inflammation, offering a gentle way to ease discomfort. Similarly, slippery elm, a supplement derived from tree bark, can protect the gut lining and improve its function. By strengthening the gut barrier, these remedies ensure your digestive system operates smoothly, keeping discomfort and imbalance at bay.

Incorporating anti-inflammatory foods into your meals doesn't have to be complicated. Consider starting your day with a berry and nut breakfast bowl, combining antioxidant-rich fruits with healthy fats for a balanced meal. For lunch or dinner, turmeric and ginger-infused dishes can add warmth and flavor while enhancing your body's defenses. These spices are delicious and packed with compounds that fight inflammation. By weaving these foods into your diet, you can enjoy meals that are both satisfying and supportive of your health.

BLOOD TYPE DIETS - PERSONALIZING YOUR NUTRITION

Picture this: a diet tailored to your blood type, promising to unlock the secrets of your body's nutritional needs. That's the allure of the blood type diet, a concept that caught many people's attention. Developed by Dr. Peter D'Adamo, this diet suggests that each blood type—A, B, AB, and O—benefits from specific foods, to optimize digestion and weight management. The idea is rooted in the belief that our ancestors' diets shaped our genetic makeup, influencing how we metabolize food today. For instance, Type O is said to thrive on a high-protein diet, while Type A does better with plant-based foods. It's a fascinating theory that connects our biology to the foods we eat.

But how does it hold up under scientific scrutiny? Research on blood type diets has been mixed, with some studies suggesting no significant benefit, while others indicate potential links to improved health markers. A study from the Toronto Nutrigenomics and Health study found some associations between blood type diets and cardiometabolic health, but these benefits weren't dependent on blood type itself. Critics argue that the diet oversimplifies human nutrition and lacks robust scientific evidence. Experts often recommend looking beyond blood type to consider genetic and metabolic profiling for more precise dietary guidance.

Personalized nutrition has gained traction by tailoring diets to individual health goals and needs. Genetic testing and metabolic profiling can provide insights into how your body processes nutrients, helping you make informed dietary choices. For those curious about personalizing their diet, starting with a food and symptom diary can be enlightening. Recording what you eat and how you feel helps identify patterns and sensitivities. Consulting with a nutritionist can offer tailored advice, ensuring your diet aligns with your unique health goals and preferences. This approach promotes a more in-depth understanding of your body's needs and can enhance your overall well-being.

CARNIVORE VS. PLANT-BASED DIETS - PROS AND CONS

Choosing the right diet can feel like navigating a labyrinth of options, each promising a healthier, more vibrant you. The carnivore diet, often called radical, centers on animal products—meat, eggs, and some dairy—and excludes plant-based foods entirely. It's rich in protein and fats, with minimal, if any, carbohydrates. Advocates argue it can lead to weight loss and improved mental clarity. However, there's a catch. Such a diet may lead to nutrient deficiencies, particularly in vitamins C and E, fiber, and specific phytonutrients, which are abundant in plants. On the other side, a plant-based diet emphasizes fruits, vegetables, grains, nuts, and seeds, offering a plethora of fiber and phytonutrients. These components support gut microbiota diversity and overall health, acting like fuel for the friendly bacteria in your gut.

The health impacts of these diets are equally varied. A carnivore diet might seem effective for weight loss due to its high protein content, which can help increase satiety and reduce overall calorie intake. However, the lack of fiber can lead to digestive issues, and a high intake of saturated fats may increase cardiovascular risks. Plant-based diets, by contrast, are often linked to lower cholesterol levels and reduced risk of chronic diseases. Their high fiber content supports digestive health and can aid in weight management by promoting fullness and regulating blood sugar levels. Yet, without careful planning, plant-based diets may lack sufficient protein and certain minerals like iron and calcium.

Our gut bacteria are remarkably adaptable and can adjust to dietary changes. A diet rich in plants can boost the production of short-chain fatty acids, known for their role in reducing inflammation and supporting metabolic health. Conversely, a diet high in animal products may decrease microbial diversity, impacting the production of these beneficial compounds. When considering which diet suits your lifestyle and goals, reflect on your nutritional needs, health objectives, and personal preferences. A balanced approach, incorporating elements from both diets, offers the flexibility and variety needed to support your gut health and overall well-being.

PALEO VS. KETO DIETS - PROS AND CONS

Paleo and keto diets have gained significant popularity, making it interesting to explore their impact on gut health.

The Paleo Diet can have both positive and negative effects on gut health, depending on how it's followed. While it emphasizes animal protein, it also includes whole, unprocessed foods such as vegetables, fruits, nuts, and seeds, which support a healthy gut microbiome. By eliminating processed foods, refined sugars, and artificial additives, the paleo diet may help reduce gut inflammation and improve digestion. However, it excludes legumes, whole grains, and dairy—key sources of prebiotics and fermentable fibers that nourish beneficial gut bacteria.

To support gut health on a paleo diet, it's essential to include a variety of fiber-rich, prebiotic foods such as onions, garlic, leeks, and asparagus, along with starchy options like cooked-and-cooled sweet potatoes and green bananas. Incorporating fermented foods like sauerkraut, kimchi, and kombucha can further promote a balanced microbiome.

The Keto Diet can have both positive and negative effects on gut health, depending on how it is followed and the individual's unique microbiome. Being low in processed sugars and refined carbohydrates, it may help reduce gut inflammation and alleviate conditions like Irritable Bowel Syndrome (IBS) and Crohn's disease. However, because it often restricts fiber-rich foods such as fruits, whole grains, and legumes—key sources of prebiotics—this can lead to dysbiosis (gut imbalance).

To support gut bacteria while following keto, it's important to include fiber-rich, low-carb vegetables like leafy greens, asparagus, and cauliflower, along with fermented foods such as sauerkraut, kimchi, and yogurt. Staying hydrated is essential to prevent constipation, while incorporating small amounts of resistant starch from green bananas, rice, or potatoes can further nourish beneficial gut bacteria.

When done properly, the keto diet can support gut health, but inadequate fiber intake may reduce microbial diversity. A well-balanced approach that includes fiber and probiotic foods is crucial for maintaining a healthy gut.

FOOD COMBINING - UNLOCKING DIGESTIVE EFFICIENCY

Imagine a dinner plate, its contents strategically arranged for flavor and optimal digestion. That's the essence of food combining, a method that organizes meals based on the belief that specific food pairings can enhance or hinder digestion. The principle is simple: avoid pairing proteins and carbohydrates in the same meal, as they require different enzymes and digestive times. Focus on eating fruits alone and on an empty stomach, allowing them to pass quickly through your system without fermenting or causing gas. The concept emphasizes meal timing, recommending that lighter foods —such as salads and fruits—be eaten first to prepare the digestive system for heavier ones, ensuring smoother digestion.

While food combining lacks robust scientific backing, its roots dig deep into history, originating in ancient Ayurvedic traditions and later popularized in the early 20th century. Despite mixed evidence from scientific studies, many individuals swear by the benefits of food combining, sharing personal tales of reduced bloating, enhanced energy, and improved digestion. It's become a topic of debate, with some experts dismissing it as pseudoscience, while others highlight the anecdotal success stories that can't be ignored. Like many dietary approaches, individual experiences vary widely, making it both intriguing and controversial.

If you're curious about food combining, start with simple steps. Eat proteins and carbohydrates at separate meals to see how your body responds. Consume proteins and vegetables at one meal, and carbohydrates and vegetables at another. Try eating fruits on an empty stomach, as a breakfast starter or a mid-morning snack. This gentle approach allows you to tune in to your body's reactions without overwhelming changes. One friend of mine, Rachel, found that switching to this method eased her persistent acid reflux, something she had battled for years with little relief from medications. Similarly, a case study I read detailed a woman's success in alleviating chronic bloating by following these principles. Both stories highlight the potential for positive change, inviting you to explore and listen to your body.

INTERMITTENT FASTING TECHNIQUES - IMPACT AND BENEFITS

The concept of intermittent fasting has been floating around wellness circles for some time now, and with good reason. At its core, intermittent fasting is about meal timing and how it can influence metabolism. It involves cycling between periods of eating and fasting, which can enhance metabolic health by allowing the body to tap into stored fat for energy during fasting periods. This approach can support weight management by encouraging the body to burn fat more efficiently rather than relying solely on the calories from recent meals. This method can also simplify meal planning, as it reduces the number of meals to prepare each day.

Fasting can have a profound effect on energy levels. While it might seem counterintuitive, many people feel more energized and mentally sharp during fasting. This is because fasting can promote the production of ketones, an alternative fuel source for the brain. Ketones can improve focus and concentration, providing a clearer mental state. However, it's important to approach fasting with flexibility, as each person's experience can differ. Some might feel fatigued initially, especially if they are used to frequent meals, but this often improves as the body adapts to the new eating pattern.

Incorporating fasting into your routine can be surprisingly straightforward. One popular method is the 16/8 approach, where you fast for 16 hours and eat during an 8-hour window. This might mean having your first meal at noon and your last by 8pm. Another option is the 5:2 method, which involves eating normally for five days and restricting calorie intake on two non-consecutive days. These methods can be adjusted to fit your lifestyle, making adopting fasting as a regular practice easier. However, listening to your body and adjusting as needed is crucial.

Despite its benefits, intermittent fasting isn't suitable for everyone. Individuals with certain medical conditions, like diabetes or eating disorders, should avoid fasting or consult a healthcare professional before starting. Pregnant or breastfeeding women should also exercise caution, as fasting might not provide the necessary nutrients during these stages. It's about finding what works for you without compromising your health.

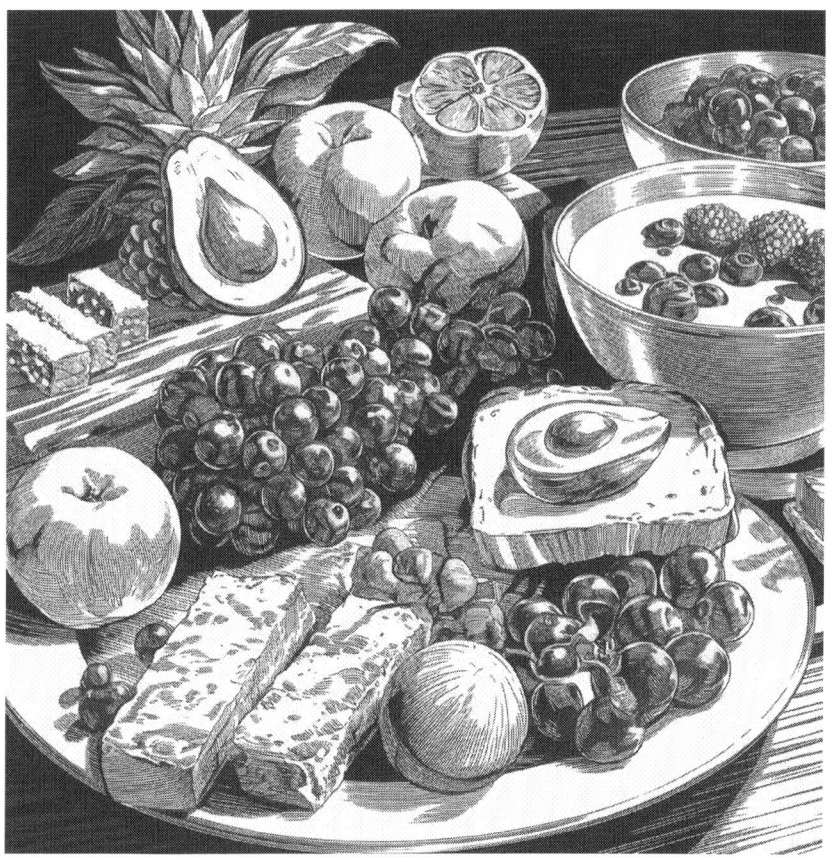

YOUR REVIEW CAN GUIDE OTHERS ON THEIR JOURNEY
TAKE A MOMENT TO SHARE YOUR THOUGHTS

"No act of kindness, no matter how small, is ever wasted."

— AESOP

As I sit here sipping a warm cup of ginger tea, I can't help but think about the journey that led me to write this book. Like you, I've searched for answers, tried countless remedies, and wondered if I'd ever feel truly at peace in my own body. If *The Gut Health Solution* has helped you in any way—maybe a little less bloating, a little more energy, or just a new understanding of what your gut really needs—I have one small favor to ask.

Would you take a moment to help someone else on this same path?

Most people pick up a book based on what others say about it. Your review could be the reason someone finally takes control of their gut health. It costs nothing, takes less than a minute, and could change the course of someone's wellness journey.

Your words might inspire...

...one more person to heal their gut.

...one more restless night to turn into deep, peaceful sleep.

...one more life to change for the better.

If you'd like to pay it forward, just scan the QR code below and leave a quick review:

"It is only through trying new things that we grow."

— UNKNOWN

7
ENERGY AND MENTAL CLARITY THROUGH DIGESTIVE HEALTH

I remember days when I felt I was just dragging, struggling to muster energy for even the simplest task. It was an overwhelming fatigue that sapped my vitality at its core. As I embarked on my journey to better gut health, I discovered a profound link between energy production and the nutrients my gut absorbed—or failed to absorb. This revelation shifted my perspective on how integral our digestive system is to maintaining energy levels and mental clarity.

The gut is pivotal in nutrient absorption and vital for energy production. Imagine the gut lining as a finely tuned conveyor belt, facilitating the transport of essential vitamins and minerals into the bloodstream. One of the key players in this process is the intestinal villi—tiny, finger-like projections that line the small intestine. These villi increase the surface area for absorption, allowing for a more efficient uptake of nutrients. When these structures are healthy, they optimize nutrient efficiency, ensuring our bodies have the necessary building blocks for energy metabolism. However, if the gut barrier is compromised, nutrient absorption can falter, leaving us feeling depleted and fatigued.

Among the myriad of nutrients absorbed through the gut, certain ones stand out for their crucial roles in energy metabolism. B vitamins are at the forefront, acting as coenzymes in converting carbohydrates, fats, and proteins into adenosine triphosphate (ATP)—the energy currency of our cells. Without adequate B vitamins, our ability to generate energy diminishes, impacting everything from physical endurance to cognitive function. Magnesium and iron also play vital roles, with magnesium involved in over 300 enzymatic reactions including energy production, and iron being essential for oxygen transport and cellular respiration. Ensuring adequate intake of these nutrients is fundamental to sustaining energy levels and supporting overall health.

Several factors can influence the efficiency of nutrient absorption in the gut. A balanced pH level in the stomach is essential, as it creates an environment conducive to activating digestive enzymes that break down food. If the pH is off-kilter, it can hinder enzyme production and nutrient uptake. Additionally, the overall health of the gut influences enzyme production. A robust gut microbiome supports optimal digestion and absorption, while imbalances can lead to inefficiencies and nutrient deficiencies. These factors underscore the importance of maintaining a healthy gut environment to enhance nutrient absorption and energy production.

Several strategies can be implemented to optimize nutrient absorption. Digestive enzyme supplements can aid in the breakdown of food, facilitating better absorption of vitamins and minerals. These supplements can benefit individuals with compromised digestive function, providing extra support to ensure proper nutrient uptake. Additionally, focusing on techniques to increase the bioavailability of nutrients can make a significant difference. For example, pairing iron-rich foods with vitamin C sources can enhance iron absorption, while soaking or sprouting grains and legumes can reduce antinutrients that inhibit nutrient uptake.

REFLECTION SECTION

Consider keeping a food journal for a week, noting any patterns between your meals and energy levels. Reflect on which foods leave you feeling energized or fatigued, and explore whether certain dietary adjustments might improve your nutrient absorption and overall vitality. This exercise can provide valuable insights into how your gut health influences your energy and mental clarity, empowering you to make informed choices that support your well-being.

GUT HEALTH AND COGNITIVE FUNCTION

I often find myself marveling at the remarkable connection between the gut and the brain. It's fascinating how the gut microbiome, this rich world of microorganisms, can influence our mental clarity and cognitive abilities. Our gut isn't just about digestion; it plays a vital role in brain function. Gut-derived neurotransmitters are at the heart of this connection. These chemical messengers, like serotonin and dopamine, travel from the gut to the brain, impacting mood and mental clarity. The vagus nerve, a significant communication line, plays a crucial role in this process. It acts as a highway, transmitting signals between the gut and brain, influencing our thoughts and feelings. This connection is a testament to the gut-brain axis, a more intertwined system than many realize.

When the microbiome is balanced, the cognitive benefits are astounding. Memory sharpens. Focus intensifies. You might recall details more easily, like remembering where you left your keys or the name of that song playing on the radio. Concentration improves, allowing you to immerse deeply in tasks. This enhancement in cognitive function is due to a well-nurtured gut environment that thrives with the right balance of bacteria. When everything is in harmony, your brain can perform at its best, making daily challenges more manageable and less draining.

On the flip side, imbalances in the gut microbiome can lead to cognitive decline. Neuroinflammation, often a result of gut issues, can impair brain function, leading to that dreaded brain fog. It's the kind of fog that makes everything seem hazy, where concentrating feels like slogging through mud. This can exacerbate difficulties in focusing or remembering things. Over time, chronic gut imbalances may even contribute to more severe neurodegenerative diseases. The links between a troubled gut and cognitive impairment highlight the importance of maintaining a healthy microbiome, not just for our physical health but also for our mental acuity.

So, how can you support your cognitive health through gut care? Start by incorporating omega-3 fatty acids into your diet. Foods like salmon or flaxseed are rich in these healthy fats, which are known to support brain health. Including B-vitamin-rich foods, such as leafy greens and whole grains, can further enhance cognitive function. These vitamins are vital for maintaining brain energy and reducing mental fatigue. Reducing sugar intake is another crucial step. High sugar levels can disrupt gut balance, impacting brain performance. Staying hydrated is equally essential, as dehydration can impair cognitive abilities, leaving you feeling sluggish.

Stress reduction techniques can also benefit the gut-brain axis. Consider simple practices like deep breathing or meditation, which calm the mind and support gut health. Avoiding excessive caffeine and alcohol can prevent disruptions in both gut and brain function. Caffeine, while a quick energy boost, can lead to jitters and disrupt sleep, affecting cognitive clarity. Alcohol, in excess, can harm the gut lining, impacting nutrient absorption and brain health. By making these small yet impactful changes, you can nurture a healthy gut environment that supports mental clarity and cognitive resilience.

It's about creating a lifestyle fostering gut and brain health, where each choice contributes to a clearer, more focused mind.

OVERCOMING FATIGUE WITH PROBIOTIC SUPERFOODS

There was a time when my afternoons felt like trudging through molasses. Energy drained away, leaving me in a foggy haze, desperate for a quick pick-me-up. That's when I stumbled upon the potential of probiotic superfoods. Fermented foods, those tangy, lively bites, are more than just culinary delights; they are natural energy boosters packed with probiotics. These foods have the remarkable ability to combat fatigue by reducing inflammation and promoting a healthy gut environment. Probiotics work within our digestive system, playing a crucial role in supporting energy levels by optimizing the efficiency of our mitochondria—the powerhouses of our cells. By enhancing mitochondrial efficiency, these friendly bacteria help us harness more energy from the nutrients we consume, turning the food we eat into the vitality we crave.

The effect of probiotics on our gut is fascinating. They reduce inflammation-related fatigue by maintaining a balanced gut microbiota, which is crucial because chronic inflammation can sap our energy reserves. Probiotics also enhance nutrient absorption, ensuring our bodies receive the full benefit of the vitamins and minerals we consume. This efficient nutrient uptake translates to more energy available for our daily activities. You might have heard of Lactobacillus reuteri, a probiotic strain known for its energy-enhancing properties. It supports the production of vitamin B12, a vital nutrient for energy metabolism. Additionally, Bifidobacterium longum can be your ally in vitality, helping to maintain a balanced gut flora that supports optimal energy levels. These strains work together to create an internal environment where fatigue is less likely to take hold, allowing you to feel more vibrant and alert.

Incorporating probiotic superfoods into your diet can be a delicious venture. Consider starting your day with a creamy kefir breakfast smoothie. Kefir, a cultured dairy product rich in probiotics, provides a refreshing start that sets a positive tone for the day. Its tartness pairs well with fruits like berries or bananas, offering a nutritious, energy-boosting meal. Another versatile option is miso, a fermented soybean paste that can enhance soups and dressings with its savory depth. A spoonful of miso dissolved in hot water creates a comforting broth, perfect for a light lunch or an afternoon pick-me-up. These foods support gut health and infuse your meals with flavors that delight the senses.

For those new to fermented foods, it's best to introduce them gradually. Much like a garden, your gut thrives with gentle care and attention. As you explore these probiotic-rich options, pay attention to how your body responds. You may notice shifts in your energy levels, along with improvements in digestion and overall well-being. Over time, these foods can become staples in your diet, offering a sustainable way to combat fatigue and boost vitality. Embrace the journey of finding which probiotic superfoods resonate with you, experimenting with different combinations and recipes to discover what makes you feel your best. Let these foods be your allies in achieving the sustained energy and vitality you deserve.

MENTAL HEALTH BENEFITS OF A BALANCED MICROBIOME

There's something incredible about how our gut and mind are connected. It's not just about digestion but how a balanced gut can lift your mood and ease those anxious days. When your gut microbiome is in harmony, it produces neurotransmitters that regulate mood. You've probably heard about serotonin, often called the "happiness hormone." A large portion of serotonin is actually produced in the gut, not the brain. This neurotransmitter plays a vital role in mood regulation and overall mental well-being. Our gut bacteria also influence the production of gamma-aminobutyric acid (GABA), which helps calm the nervous system and provides a sense of relaxation. By nurturing a healthy gut environment, you're supporting the production of these mood-regulating chemicals, which can alleviate symptoms of anxiety and depression.

The benefits of a balanced microbiome extend beyond individual neurotransmitters. With robust gut health, you may notice reduced anxiety levels and improved emotional stability. Stressful situations that once seemed overwhelming might feel more manageable. This resilience to stress is partly due to the gut's influence on the stress response system. A well-balanced microbiome can help regulate cortisol, the body's primary stress hormone, keeping it in check. By doing so, it allows you to navigate life's challenges with a steadier, calmer mindset. This doesn't mean stress magically disappears, but rather your body becomes better equipped to handle it, like having a safety net ready to catch you when needed.

The gut's ability to produce neurotransmitters is a fascinating process. Besides serotonin, it also influences dopamine production. Dopamine is crucial for motivation, pleasure, and reward. Imagine finding joy in activities that once felt mundane, or regaining the drive to pursue your passions. These neurotransmitters work together to maintain a balanced mood and enhance your emotional well-being. The interplay between the gut and brain is a reminder that caring for your digestive health isn't just about physical comfort; it's about nurturing your mental health as well. A thriving microbiome can lead to a more balanced, fulfilling life, where you feel more in tune with your emotions and more capable of handling life's ups and downs.

To maintain a microbiome that supports mental health, consider incorporating certain practices into your routine. Start by adding prebiotic-rich foods like garlic, onions, and bananas to your diet.

These foods fuel the beneficial bacteria in your gut, promoting a healthy environment for neurotransmitter production. Regular physical activity can also support gut health. Exercise stimulates the release of endorphins, which are natural mood elevators, and enhances gut motility, helping maintain a balanced microbiome. Incorporating yoga into your routine can further reduce stress and support gut health. The mindful movements and deep breathing in yoga can lower cortisol levels, promoting relaxation and mental clarity. These practices work together to create a supportive environment for both your gut and mind, offering a holistic approach to well-being.

Our mental health is intricately linked to our gut health. The two work in tandem, influencing how we feel and react to the world around us. By taking steps to support a balanced microbiome, you're not just aiding your digestion but fostering a more resilient, balanced, and emotionally stable version of yourself. As we explore these connections, it becomes clear that the path to mental wellness is paved with mindful, gut-friendly choices that empower you to live a more vibrant, fulfilling life.

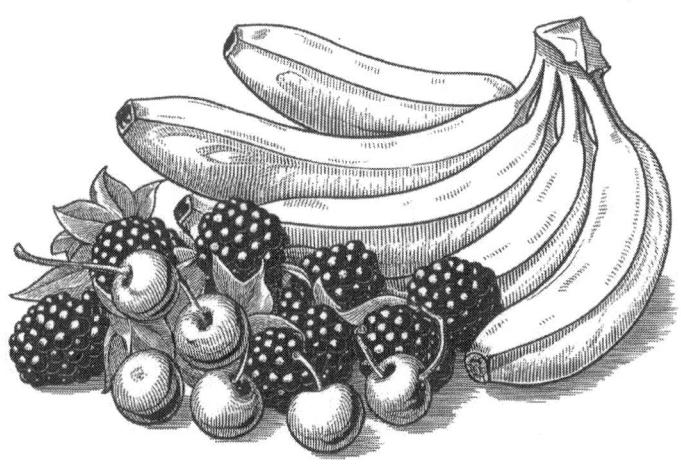

8

INTEGRATING INNOVATION AND TECHNOLOGY

It's incredible how technology has integrated into every aspect of our lives, constantly providing innovative solutions and introducing new advancements on a daily basis. I've spent countless hours jotting down notes about my digestive health, trying to piece together patterns and triggers. But let's be honest—keeping track of everything with pen and paper can be a bit of a chore. Enter the world of digital health tracking. Imagine having a tool that organizes all those scribbles and transforms them into meaningful insights. That's the magic of gut health tracking apps. They're like your personal detective and secretary, tirelessly gathering and organizing clues to help you solve the mystery of your gut.

There are a growing number of apps dedicated to gut health, each with its own set of features designed to make the process as seamless as possible. Take *Plop*, for example, which offers a unique approach by tracking bowel movements, giving you a visual snapshot of your digestive health. Or consider *Bowelle*, which goes a step further by allowing you to log food intake, symptoms, water consumption, and even stress levels. These tools offer a holistic view of your health, helping you see how different factors interplay to affect your gut. Using such apps is like having a pocket-sized health advisor who listens and learns from your daily experiences and gives you feedback.

The core benefit of these technological tools lies in their ability to collect real-time data. Rather than waiting for a doctor's appointment to discuss your symptoms, you can have immediate feedback. This empowers you to make informed decisions and helps you swiftly identify patterns and triggers. Imagine noticing that a particular food consistently causes discomfort—having that insight can help you make adjustments before issues escalate. It's like having a dashboard for your digestive health that lets you steer your wellness journey with precision and confidence.

When choosing the right app, finding one that fits seamlessly into your lifestyle is essential. User-friendly interfaces are key—after all, the last thing you want is to spend hours figuring out an app. Look for customization options that let you tailor the app to focus on what's most relevant to you. Some apps, like *Low FODMAP diet A to Z*, offer expert recommendations and community support, providing a sense of reassurance and connection. This can be particularly valuable if you're starting to explore dietary changes or need guidance along the way. It's about finding a tool that feels like an extension of yourself, reflecting your unique needs and preferences.

REFLECTION SECTION

Take a moment to consider what you'd like to achieve with a gut health app. Is it tracking symptoms, logging meals, or finding community support? Write down your goals and priorities. This will guide you in selecting an app that aligns with your health objectives. Remember, the right tool can be a valuable ally, helping you unlock insights and take control of your gut health journey.

ONLINE COMMUNITIES AND SUPPORT NETWORKS

Online communities have emerged as vibrant meeting spaces for those navigating the complexities of gut health. Often found on forums and in social media groups, these serve as gathering places for individuals seeking camaraderie and understanding. When I first ventured into these communities, I was struck by the sense of solidarity and shared purpose. There were people exchanging stories that resonated with my experiences, revealing the universal challenge of managing digestive issues. It was like finding a supportive tribe that understood the nuanced journey of gut health, offering me a chance to learn from the insights and experiences of others.

Peer support within these communities is invaluable. It provides a sense of connection and belonging, especially when you feel isolated by your symptoms. Engaging with others who face similar challenges enhances motivation and adherence to gut health goals. It's encouraging to see members offer emotional support and practical advice, from dietary tips to stress management techniques. The exchange of strategies is like a collective brainstorming session, sparking new ideas and approaches. There's also an element of accountability; knowing that others are cheering for your success can make all the difference to sticking to a diet when you're about to backslide. It transforms the solitary health journey into a collaborative effort where everyone's progress is celebrated and acknowledged.

Yet, amidst the wealth of information, caution is necessary. The internet is a double-edged sword, where credible advice often sits alongside misinformation. It's crucial to approach online health information critically, evaluating the quality and accuracy of what's shared. Recognizing credible sources and experts is key; look for evidence-based recommendations and insights from healthcare professionals. Avoid unverified claims or anecdotal advice presented as fact, as these can lead to confusion or misguided decisions. Think of it as sifting through a treasure trove—there are gems to be found, but they require discernment and careful consideration.

Actively engaging in online communities can be a rewarding endeavor. Start by sharing your experiences and success stories, offering a glimpse into your unique journey with gut health. This fosters connection and encourages others to open up about their challenges and triumphs. Asking questions and seeking advice from community members can provide diverse perspectives and solutions you might not have considered. It's a dynamic exchange of knowledge and support where everyone has something to offer. Remember, the goal is to contribute positively and constructively, creating an environment where everyone feels valued and heard.

REFLECTION SECTION

Consider joining an online gut health community if you haven't already done so. Reflect on what you want to gain from this experience, whether it's support, information, or simply a sense of belonging. Write a few thoughts about your goals and how you plan to engage with others. This reflection can guide your interactions and help you maximize your time in these virtual spaces.

INTERACTIVE QUIZZES FOR PERSONALIZED GUT HEALTH PLANS

Reflecting on the endless options available for gut health, I gravitated toward interactive quizzes. They act like a compass, guiding you through the maze of health information to zero in on what truly matters to you. Imagine sitting down with a virtual health coach who asks all the right questions about your eating habits, stress levels, and even symptoms that seem to appear out of nowhere. These quizzes dive deep into your health profile, offering insights to help you understand your body's unique needs. Whether you're using them through an app or an online platform, these quizzes provide a personalized touch, making your wellness journey less about guesswork and more about informed decisions.

The beauty of these quizzes lies in their ability to offer personalized recommendations based on your responses and craft a plan as individual as your fingerprint. A well-designed quiz can highlight potential food sensitivities or imbalances. It may suggest cutting back on dairy or increasing your fiber intake. Or it could identify a need for stress management techniques to help calm your gut. These quizzes evaluate symptoms and their severity, giving you a clearer picture of what's happening inside your body. Armed with this information, you can make informed choices about your diet and lifestyle, tailoring them to support your gut health effectively.

Several platforms offer reputable gut health quizzes, each with its unique approach and methodology. For example, take a look at *Complement's* personalized nutrition quiz. This platform stands out by integrating professional healthcare advice from medical doctors and registered dietitians, ensuring the recommendations you receive are grounded in science. User testimonials and high ratings provide an added layer of trust, reflecting the positive experiences of others who have embarked on a similar health exploration. As you explore these quizzes, it's important to remember that they are tools to guide you, not a replacement for professional medical advice. Their strength lies in their ability to offer a starting point, a direction to explore further with the help of healthcare professionals.

The potential of interactive quizzes extends beyond simple assessments. They can be a stepping stone toward a more proactive approach to your health. By identifying specific areas that require attention, these quizzes empower you to take control of your wellbeing. They can suggest dietary adjustments, recommend lifestyle changes, and even highlight areas for further investigation with a healthcare provider. It's like having a personalized roadmap that adapts to your needs, helping you confidently navigate the complexities of gut health. As you engage with these quizzes, you'll likely discover insights that resonate with your experiences, opening doors to further possibilities for a healthier, more balanced life.

In the ever-evolving landscape of health and wellness, interactive quizzes offer a unique opportunity to actively engage with your gut health journey. They invite you to participate actively in your well-being, encouraging self-reflection and informed decision-making. As you embrace the insights and recommendations these quizzes provide, they will help you become better equipped to make choices supporting your gut health and overall vitality.

UTILIZING QR CODES FOR EXCLUSIVE CONTENT ACCESS

QR codes have become an unexpected ally in our quest for better health. These little squares might seem unassuming at first, but they pack a powerful punch when it comes to accessing a treasure trove of health resources. The beauty of QR codes lies in their simplicity and efficiency. With a quick scan using your smartphone, you're instantly transported to a world of exclusive content designed to enhance your understanding of gut health. This can range from insightful videos and articles to interviews with experts who shed light on complex topics. Imagine standing in your kitchen, wondering how to incorporate more fermented foods into your diet, and with a swift scan, you're watching a chef demonstrate a step-by-step recipe. It's like having a personal health library in your pocket, ready to offer guidance whenever needed.

The interactive nature of content delivered through QR codes is what makes it so engaging. Instead of passively reading an article, you can immerse yourself in a dynamic learning experience. Visual learners can benefit from videos demonstrating techniques, while auditory learners may appreciate podcasts or guided meditations to reduce stress, a known trigger for gut issues. This multimedia approach caters to diverse learning styles, making the information more accessible and easier to retain. It's a way to keep the content fresh and exciting, ensuring that you're informed and inspired to take action. This kind of engagement can transform how you approach your gut health journey, turning it into an interactive adventure rather than a solitary chore.

You can access countless types of exclusive content through QR codes, each adding a new dimension to your understanding of gut health. Picture scanning a code and being led to an expert Q&A session where specialists answer burning questions about probiotics or the impact of stress on digestion. Or you may need a moment of calm, and a quick scan offers a guided meditation session designed to soothe your mind and body. These resources provide practical insights and techniques that you can immediately integrate into your daily life. It's like having a toolkit of knowledge at your fingertips, ready to support you in your health endeavors.

Incorporating QR codes into your daily routine can be seamless and rewarding. Consider scanning codes during meal preparation to access recipe guidance, ensuring your meals are delicious and supportive of gut health. Use codes to receive daily wellness tips and affirmations, helping you start your day with a positive mindset. By making QR codes a regular part of your routine, you open yourself up to continuous learning and support, reinforcing your commitment to a healthier lifestyle. It's about creating an environment where knowledge is always within reach, empowering you to make informed decisions.

The integration of QR codes into health and wellness represents a step forward in how we access and engage with information. They offer a unique way to connect with content that is both informative and motivational, creating a richer, more interactive experience. As we continue exploring the possibilities of technology in health, QR codes stand out as a versatile tool that enhances our ability to learn, grow, and thrive. In the next chapter, we'll shift our focus to cost-effective solutions for gut health, exploring practical strategies to maintain balance without breaking the bank. This chapter has laid the groundwork for understanding the role of technology in health, setting the stage for the practical applications that follow.

9
COST-EFFECTIVE SOLUTIONS FOR GUT HEALTH

Have you ever stood in the grocery aisle, contemplating the cost of a health food product that promises to transform your gut health, only to put it back on the shelf because it wasn't in the budget? I have many times. The world of gut health is filled with enticing options, but they often come with a hefty price tag. This chapter is all about finding those hidden gems—cost-effective solutions that safeguard your digestive health without breaking the bank. One of the most straightforward and rewarding approaches is embracing the art of fermenting foods at home. This practice is budget-friendly and unlocks a treasure trove of health benefits that commercially made alternatives can't consistently deliver.

When you make your own fermented foods, you're engaging in a process that has been cherished for centuries. Fermentation extends the shelf life of foods and enhances their nutritional value, providing a boost of probiotics essential for healthy digestion. Unlike many store-bought options, which contain added sugars or lack live cultures due to pasteurization, homemade fermentations are full of life. By nurturing the growth of beneficial bacteria, you support your gut microbiome, which plays a critical role in digestion, immune function, and even mental clarity. It's like turning your kitchen into a mini-laboratory, where science and tradition combine to create something genuinely nourishing.

The beauty of home fermentation lies in its simplicity and affordability. All you need to get started are a few basic tools and ingredients. First, you'll want some glass jars—Mason jars work perfectly—as they allow you to monitor your progress. Though not essential, fermentation weights can help keep veggies submerged under the brine, preventing spoilage. Depending on the recipe, you might use natural sea salt to create a brine, and live starter cultures, like whey or a scoop of yogurt, to kick-start the process. Vegetables such as cabbage for sauerkraut or cucumbers for pickles are readily available and inexpensive, making them ideal candidates for fermentation experiments. The best part? You get to control every ingredient, ensuring your products are as natural and healthful as possible.

Safety and hygiene are paramount when fermenting at home. The last thing you want is to spend time and effort only to end up with a batch that's gone bad. Start by sterilizing your jars and equipment. This can be done by washing them in hot, soapy water and letting them air-dry completely. When preparing your ingredients, maintain a clean workspace to prevent contamination. Over time, watch for signs of successful fermentation, such as bubbling and a tangy aroma. These indicate that beneficial bacteria are hard at work. If you notice any off smells or mold, it's best to discard the batch and start anew. Remember, patience is key. Fermentation is a slow but rewarding process, and the results are well worth the wait.

FERMENTATION CHECKLIST

- **Glass Jars:** Ensure they are clean and sterilized before use.

- **Fermentation Weights:** Optional, but helpful for keeping vegetables submerged.
- **Natural Sea Salt:** Essential for creating a brine.
- **Live Starter Cultures:** Use whey or yogurt for added probiotics.
- **Clean Workspace:** Maintain hygiene to prevent contamination.
- **Monitor Progress:** Look for bubbling and a tangy aroma as signs of success.

Incorporating these practices into your routine not only empowers you to take charge of your gut health but also offers a deeper connection to the foods you consume. There's something profoundly satisfying about savoring a crisp, homemade pickle, knowing it's a delicious testament to your own efforts. Fermentation is more than a cooking method; it's a celebration of patience, tradition, and the incredible potential of nature to nurture us.

BUDGET-FRIENDLY SUPERFOODS FOR DIGESTIVE WELLNESS

Superfoods often carry an air of exclusivity, conjuring images of exotic powders and pricey supplements. Yet, some of the most potent superfoods for gut health are humble and accessible, hiding on your grocery store shelves in plain sight. Take oats, for instance. These unassuming grains are a powerhouse of beta-glucan, a soluble fiber that supports cholesterol management and digestion. Incorporating oats into your diet can help maintain healthy blood sugar levels and keep your digestive tract moving smoothly. The versatility of oats is a bonus, allowing you to enjoy them in countless forms, from overnight oats to hearty oat-based soups.

Chia seeds, another budget-friendly gem, pack a surprising punch for their size. Known for their high omega-3 fatty acid content, chia seeds are an excellent source of fiber, aiding both digestion and heart health. When soaked, they expand and form a gel-like consistency, which can help regulate bowel movements and support a healthy gut. A simple chia seed pudding, made by mixing these tiny seeds with almond milk and letting them soak overnight, offers a delightful, nutrient-dense start to your day. The beauty of chia seeds lies in their ability to blend seamlessly into smoothies, yogurts, and baked goods, making it easy to boost your nutrient intake without much effort.

Then there's the often-overlooked sweet potato, a nutritional powerhouse that deserves a spot in your pantry. Rich in vitamins, minerals, and antioxidants, sweet potatoes are also an excellent source of prebiotic fiber. Baking a sweet potato and topping it with a sprinkle of cinnamon is a simple, satisfying way to enjoy this vibrant vegetable. The sweet potato's natural sweetness and versatility make it a favorite in savory and sweet dishes, offering a comforting, nutritious option for any meal.

Shopping wisely for these superfoods can further enhance their affordability. Buying in bulk is a smart strategy, whether you're purchasing oats, chia seeds, or sweet potatoes. Local co-ops and online retailers often offer bulk discounts, allowing you to stock up and save. Prioritizing whole, unprocessed foods benefits your wallet and ensures your gut receives the nutrients it craves. Legumes and beans, another economical protein source, pair well with these superfoods to create balanced, filling meals. A visit to your local farmers' market can be an enjoyable way to find in-season produce at a lower cost, supporting your community and your gut. Choosing produce when it's in season maximizes flavor and reduces costs, making it a win-win for your budget and taste buds.

Consider starting your day with overnight oats, a quick and easy recipe that combines oats, chia seeds, and your favorite berries. Mix the ingredients, let them soak in the fridge overnight, and wake up to a ready-to-eat breakfast. For lunch or dinner, whip up a sweet potato and black bean chili. The hearty combination of sweet potatoes and beans provides fiber, protein, and a satisfying warmth, perfect for any season. These simple recipes are delicious and showcase the power of budget-friendly superfoods to elevate your gut health. By embracing these affordable options, you can nourish your body and support your digestive wellness without straining your finances.

MEAL PLANNING AND PREPARATION ON A BUDGET

Imagine a kitchen where every meal is a well-orchestrated symphony, ingredients are used to their fullest potential, and waste is minimal. That's the magic of meal planning. It's not just about saving money, though that's a significant perk. It's about creating a harmonious relationship between your diet, health, and wallet. By planning meals around sales and seasonal produce, you can enjoy a variety of fresh, nutrient-dense foods without overspending. Seasonal fruits and vegetables are cheaper and taste better, making them perfect for your meal prep. When you plan your meals, you can also reduce impulse buys, often leading to processed foods sneaking into your cart. This approach benefits your gut and keeps your spending in check.

To get started, consider creating a weekly menu based on the ingredients you already have. This prevents waste and sparks creativity in the kitchen. Look at what's in your pantry and fridge, and consider how to transform those items into delicious meals. A can of chickpeas and some leftover spinach could become a hearty stew. Utilizing leftovers is another fantastic strategy. A roast chicken could become a nourishing broth for soup or a filling for tacos. By embracing leftover transformation, you stretch your grocery budget and enjoy a variety of meals without extra cost.

In the realm of meal prep, versatility is your best friend. Grains like rice and quinoa serve as excellent bases for many dishes. They're affordable, easy to cook, and can be elevated with different herbs, spices, and toppings to keep things interesting. Incorporate versatile proteins like beans and lentils, which are cost-effective and pack a punch of nutrition. These ingredients can be used in soups, salads, or even blended into burgers. Growing herbs or small vegetables at home can enhance your meals and reduce costs. Imagine plucking fresh basil or mint from your windowsill garden to brighten your dishes.

When it comes to meal preparation, efficiency is key. Using reusable glass containers for storage is not only environmentally friendly but also practical. They keep food fresh and visible, making it easy to grab what you need. Consider batch cooking, where you prepare larger meals and freeze portions for later use. This saves time during busy weeks and ensures you always have a healthy option available. Prepping ingredients in advance can also streamline your cooking process. Chop vegetables, marinate proteins, or measure spices on a free afternoon, so everything is ready to go when it's time to cook. Planning and preparation allow you to whip up meals quickly, reducing the temptation to order takeout after a long day.

Meal planning might initially sound daunting, but it becomes second nature with practice. Start by planning a few meals a week, gradually expanding as you get comfortable. Use tools like calendars or meal-planning apps to keep track of your menu and shopping list. Involve the whole family by asking for input and preferences, turning meal planning into a collaborative effort. By making these simple yet impactful changes, you'll find that eating well on a budget is possible and deeply satisfying. The time and effort you invest in planning will pay off in delicious, gut-friendly meals supporting your health and financial goals.

DIY REMEDIES FOR COMMON DIGESTIVE COMPLAINTS

In the realm of digestive health, sometimes the simplest solutions are the most effective. Our kitchens are often stocked with ingredients that double as natural remedies, waiting to soothe minor digestive woes without the need for a pharmacy visit. Ginger, for instance, is a staple in many homes and holds a special place in my heart—and stomach—for its ability to quell nausea and ease indigestion. A warm cup of ginger tea, made by steeping fresh slices in hot water, can work wonders on an upset stomach. The spicy warmth of ginger comforts and stimulates digestion, helping to move things along when your gut feels sluggish. It's a small ritual that can bring immense relief, whether you've overindulged at dinner or need a digestive reset.

Licorice root is another ally in the battle against digestive discomfort. Known for its sweet flavor and soothing properties, licorice root has been used for centuries to support digestion. It can help protect the mucous lining of the stomach and intestines, making it particularly useful for those suffering from heartburn or ulcers. A simple licorice tea brewed with dried root can offer a gentle, sweet respite for your digestive system. However, it's important to note that not all licorice products are created equal. Look for deglycyrrhizinated licorice (DGL) if you're concerned about potential blood pressure effects, as it removes the compound responsible for these issues while retaining the digestive benefits.

With its fresh, cooling aroma, peppermint tea is a go-to for alleviating digestive discomfort. The menthol in peppermint acts as a natural muscle relaxant, soothing the gastrointestinal tract muscles. This can help relieve bloating and gas, making it a comforting choice after a meal. A steeped cup of peppermint tea refreshes the senses and calms the belly. However, if you suffer from acid reflux, it's best to approach peppermint with caution, as it can sometimes exacerbate symptoms. Peppermint tea can be a delightful and effective way to maintain digestive harmony for those who can tolerate it.

Then there's apple cider vinegar, a powerful tonic many swear by for its digestive benefits. Its acidity can help stimulate stomach acid production, aiding in the breakdown of food and smoothing the digestive process. Mixing a tablespoon of apple cider vinegar with a glass of water and sipping it before a meal can prepare your stomach for digestion. While its taste might be an acquired one, the benefits are clear. Just be sure to dilute it properly to avoid any potential acid damage to your teeth. A straw can also help mitigate contact with your enamel, preserving your smile while you nurture your gut.

These DIY remedies offer a comforting sense of control over your digestive health, empowering you to address minor complaints with ingredients you likely already have. They remind us that our kitchens are not just places for preparing meals, but spaces for healing and nurturing our bodies. Each of these remedies carries a legacy of traditional use, connecting us to generations who have relied on nature's pharmacy for relief. By incorporating these simple solutions into your routine, you can cultivate a more balanced and resilient digestive system, all while embracing the timeless wisdom of natural remedies.

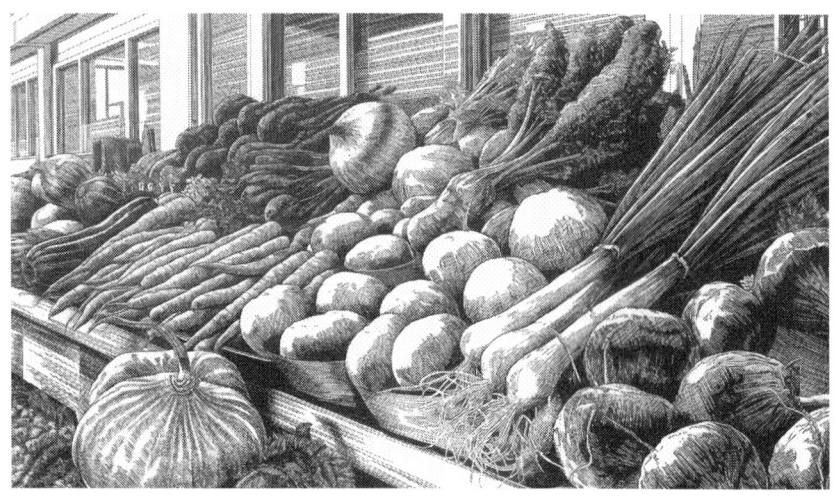

10

REAL-LIFE SUCCESS STORIES AND TESTIMONIALS

We've all been there, haven't we? Sitting in a doctor's office, feeling like your symptoms are being brushed off as "just stress", or hearing, "try cutting out dairy" as the one-size-fits-all piece of advice. It's frustrating when your health feels like a puzzle no one can solve. In these moments of exasperation, real-life stories of transformation can reignite hope and inspire change. In this chapter, I want to share stories that serve as beacons of hope, illuminating the path ahead. These are tales of real people who have transformed their gut health and overall well-being through diet, lifestyle changes, and sheer determination.

Take, for instance, a woman named Emily. For years, she wrestled with IBS, a condition that left her feeling trapped and controlled by her unpredictable digestive system. Every meal felt like a gamble. Emily's breakthrough came when she embraced a low-FODMAP diet, a targeted approach that involved eliminating certain fermentable carbs known to trigger her symptoms. The change wasn't overnight, but slowly, she began noticing fewer flare-ups and more freedom in her daily life. Alongside dietary adjustments, Emily incorporated yoga and mindfulness into her routine to help manage stress, which she recognized as a key trigger for her IBS. The combination of these changes didn't just improve her physical health—it gave her the confidence to engage socially without fear of her symptoms hijacking the moment.

Then there's Mark, who faced the daunting challenge of leaky gut syndrome. The constant fatigue and brain fog had become unwelcome companions in his life, making each day feel like a battle. Mark decided to overhaul his lifestyle, starting with an anti-inflammatory diet focused on whole, unprocessed foods. He added supplements like L-glutamine and probiotics to support his gut lining and microbiome. But it wasn't just about food; Mark found solace and healing in acupuncture, which helped balance his system and promote relaxation. Over time, the fog lifted, and so did his spirits. Mark's story is one of persistence and willingness to explore both conventional and alternative therapies to regain his health.

These stories highlight the diversity of paths taken to achieve gut health. While the low-FODMAP diet was Emily's lifeline, Mark's journey was about finding the right mix of dietary changes and complementary therapies. The personalized nature of these approaches underscores the importance of listening to one's body and being open to trying different strategies. Whether it's the Autoimmune Protocol (AIP) diet or integrating practices like acupuncture and yoga, the key is finding what resonates with you and your unique circumstances.

Beyond the physical transformations, the emotional and psychological impacts are profound. Many individuals, like Emily and Mark, report significant improvements in their mental well-being alongside their gut health. Common themes include reduced anxiety, enhanced mood, and a renewed sense of joy in social interactions. It's as if lifting the burden of digestive distress also lifts the veil of emotional heaviness. For Emily, the ability to dine out with friends without the looming fear of an IBS attack brought back a sense of normalcy and happiness. Reclaiming mental clarity allowed Mark to engage more fully in his work and personal life, rekindling his zest for living.

The journeys of these individuals offer valuable insights and practical tips that can inspire your own path to better health. Patience and persistence are crucial, as is the willingness to seek professional guidance and support. Whether it's a dietitian, a therapist, or a supportive community, having a network can make the journey less daunting and more rewarding. These stories remind us that while the road to gut health may be long and winding, it is navigable, especially when we take it one step at a time.

REFLECTION SECTION

Consider reflecting on your own health journey. What changes have you tried, and what have you learned about your body along the way? This reflection can help you identify areas where you might want to experiment with new approaches or seek additional support. Write down a few thoughts and consider discussing them with a healthcare professional or a supportive friend.

CASE STUDIES - OVERCOMING CHRONIC GUT ISSUES

One of the most challenging gut issues many people face is chronic bloating, often accompanied by a Small Intestinal Bacterial Overgrowth (SIBO) diagnosis. Consider Sarah, a determined woman who battled this uncomfortable condition for years. Her days were filled with discomfort and self-consciousness. She sought help and began her diagnostic journey with comprehensive testing, including breath tests to confirm SIBO. The results were eye-opening, revealing an overgrowth of bacteria in her small intestine. With this knowledge, Sarah's healthcare team, including a gastroenterologist and a nutritionist, crafted a personalized treatment plan. This plan focused on dietary changes, specifically a low-FODMAP diet, alongside herbals like oregano oil to target the bacterial imbalance. Continuous monitoring and adjustments were key, allowing Sarah to slowly but surely reclaim her comfort and confidence.

Another compelling case is that of Michael, who struggled with candida overgrowth. This imbalance in his gut flora led to persistent issues like fatigue, brain fog, and yeast infections. After a thorough assessment that included stool tests and consultations with a naturopath, Michael embarked on a path of targeted treatment. His regimen included a strict anti-candida diet, eliminating sugar and refined carbs, which feed the yeast. He also introduced probiotics and antifungal supplements to help restore balance. With the support of his healthcare team, Michael followed a personalized plan that was carefully monitored and adjusted as needed. Over time, he noticed a significant reduction in symptoms along with an increase in energy levels, allowing him to engage more fully in life.

These case studies underscore the importance of a multidisciplinary approach in managing chronic gut issues. Sarah and Michael's successes were not achieved in isolation but through collaboration among healthcare professionals. By integrating the expertise of gastroenterologists, nutritionists, and naturopaths, they received comprehensive care that addressed the root causes of their conditions. This team-based approach allowed for a more holistic understanding of their health, ensuring that all aspects of their well-being were considered. Personalized treatment plans tailored to their unique needs were continuously adapted based on their progress and responses. This adaptability allowed for adjustments aligned with their evolving health status and goals.

The lessons learned from these case studies are invaluable for anyone facing similar challenges. First, the importance of holistic and integrative care cannot be overstated. Combining conventional and alternative treatments offers a more rounded approach to health, addressing not just symptoms but underlying causes. Second, individualized treatment plans are key. What works for one person may not work for another, highlighting the need for personalized strategies that consider each individual's circumstances and health history. Lastly, the journey to overcoming chronic gut issues requires ongoing adaptation. As Sarah and Michael's stories illustrate, continuous monitoring and a willingness to make necessary changes are essential for achieving and maintaining health improvements.

These insights remind us that while the path to gut health may be complex, it is navigable with the right support and strategies. By embracing a comprehensive, personalized approach and working closely with a team of healthcare professionals, individuals can find relief from chronic gut issues and experience a renewed sense of well-being.

TESTIMONIALS - THE IMPACT OF LIFESTYLE CHANGES

In gut health, lifestyle changes can be transformative, often turning the tide on chronic issues that have lingered for years. Take the story of Lisa, an accountant who decided to adopt a plant-based diet after years of digestive distress. Initially skeptical, Lisa hesitated to give up her beloved dairy and meat. However, the persistent bloating and frequent stomach pains pushed her to explore new dietary avenues. With the encouragement of a friend who had successfully transitioned to a plant-based lifestyle, Lisa took the plunge. She slowly incorporated more fruits, vegetables, and whole grains into her meals while gradually reducing animal products. To her delight, Lisa noticed a reduction in her symptoms within weeks. Her digestion improved, and she felt lighter and more energetic. The shift brought physical relief and fostered a sense of empowerment as she took control of her health.

For many, lifestyle changes extend beyond diet. Consider Tom, a teacher who found solace in regular exercise and mindfulness practices. Struggling with stress-induced digestive issues, Tom decided to incorporate daily walks and meditation into his routine. At first, he faced the usual barriers—time constraints and skepticism about the effectiveness of such activities. However, his persistence paid off. Combining physical activity and mindful breathing helped alleviate his digestive discomfort and significantly reduced his stress. Tom's experience highlights the interconnectedness of mental and physical health, illustrating how addressing one can positively impact the other.

The motivations behind these lifestyle changes are varied, often rooted in a deep desire for relief and improved quality of life. Lisa's initial resistance stemmed from a fear of change and a belief that her symptoms were something she had to live with. However, her friend's success story was a ray of hope, showing her that change was possible. On the other hand, Tom was driven by a need to find balance and peace in his hectic life. Both faced challenges along the way—the initial struggle to adapt to new habits, the occasional relapse into old eating patterns, or the temptation to skip a workout. Yet, the support of friends and community groups played a crucial role in sustaining their motivation, providing encouragement and accountability when they needed it most.

The long-term benefits of these lifestyle modifications are undeniable. Lisa experienced sustained weight loss and newfound energy levels, which enhanced her overall well-being. Her journey underscores the sustainability of plant-based diets when approached with flexibility and a focus on whole, nutrient-dense foods. Meanwhile, Tom found that regular exercise and mindfulness brought lasting mental clarity and emotional stability. The practices became a cornerstone of his daily life, offering relief from digestive issues and a renewed sense of purpose and calm.

From these testimonials, practical advice emerges that can guide others on similar paths. Start small. Gradual changes allow your body and mind to adjust, reducing the likelihood of feeling overwhelmed or defeated. Lisa's gradual shift to a plant-based diet exemplifies the power of incremental change—substituting a few meals each week rather than overhauling her diet overnight. Maintaining motivation is crucial, and finding a supportive community, whether online or in person, can provide the encouragement needed to stay the course. For Tom, joining a local walking group offered companionship and accountability, making exercise a social and enjoyable activity.

Ultimately, these stories remind us that lifestyle changes are profoundly personal and should be tailored to fit individual preferences and needs. It's about finding what resonates with you, experimenting with different approaches, and being open to the possibilities that come with change. Listening to your body and honoring its signals is key, allowing you to create a sustainable path to improved gut health and overall wellness.

LESSONS LEARNED - KEY TAKEAWAYS FROM SUCCESS STORIES

As we weave through these stories of transformation, perseverance shines as a common thread. Each person faced challenges, yet they continued to push forward, adapting to ever-changing circumstances. Perseverance doesn't mean always knowing the path ahead —it's about remaining committed even when the destination is unclear. Adaptability is equally essential, allowing one to pivot and reassess strategies as new information and experiences unfold. Listening to one's body and intuition becomes a guiding compass, teaching us to recognize what our bodies need and when to make changes. These success stories remind us that our health journey is not about perfection but progress and learning to tune into our body's cues.

Community and support networks emerge as vital components in these narratives. Whether it's a friend offering encouragement or an online forum filled with like-minded individuals, these connections provide a web of support that makes the journey less lonely. Online support groups and forums offer a platform for sharing experiences and advice, fostering a sense of belonging and mutual understanding. The influence of friends and family cannot be understated. Their support often serves as a lifeline, helping individuals stay motivated and accountable. When your energy wanes, or doubt creeps in, knowing that others believe in your potential can reignite your determination and keep you moving forward.

Taking charge of one's health leads to empowerment and self-efficacy. As individuals learn more about their bodies and health conditions, they build confidence in their ability to manage their wellbeing. Knowledge becomes a powerful tool, enabling them to make informed decisions about their health. This empowerment fosters a proactive approach to health and wellness, where individuals take initiative and responsibility for their choices. They are no longer passive recipients of care; they have become active participants in their health journey, setting goals and taking steps to achieve them. This shift in mindset transforms challenges into opportunities for growth and learning.

Setting realistic goals is a crucial first step for those ready to start their own path to improved gut health. Break down larger goals into manageable actions, celebrating small victories along the way. Tracking progress can provide valuable insights and motivation, helping you see how far you've come and what adjustments might be needed. Seeking professional guidance is also important. Health professionals can offer tailored advice and resources, ensuring your strategies align with your unique needs and circumstances. Remember, it's okay to ask for help and to lean on the expertise of others as you navigate your health journey.

As we close this chapter, it's clear that the journey toward gut health is deeply personal, shaped by the interconnectedness of our bodies, minds, and communities. The stories shared here remind us of the potential for transformation when we embrace perseverance, adaptability, and self-care. We can find empowerment and confidence in managing our health through community support and a proactive approach. The lessons learned from these success stories serve as a testament to the resilience and strength within each of us, encouraging us to explore new paths and possibilities in our pursuit of wellness.

In the next chapter, we'll dive into practical strategies and recipes that can support your ongoing journey to gut health. These tools will provide a foundation for nourishing your body and mind, empowering you to continue building a vibrant and balanced life.

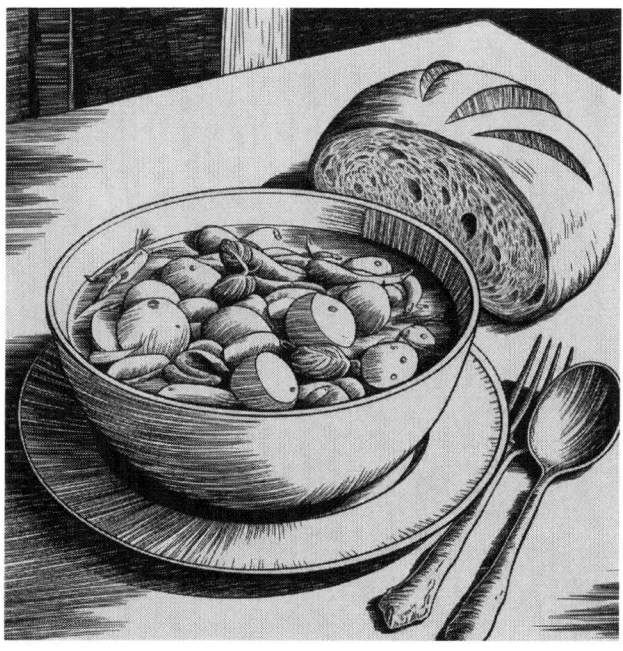

"Success is a series of small wins."

— UNKNOWN

11
RECIPES AND MEAL PLANS FOR GUT HEALTH

Cooking has always been a comforting ritual—moving through the kitchen, crafting flavorful dishes, and immersing myself in rich aromas that ground me in the moment. As someone who's spent years untangling the intricacies of gut health, I've come to appreciate the power and simplicity of homemade probiotic foods. These recipes offer a way to infuse meals with beneficial bacteria, transforming ordinary ingredients into gut-nourishing staples. When I began exploring probiotic recipes, I was pleasantly surprised by how uncomplicated they were. With just a few ingredients and a bit of patience, you can create foods that delight the palate and support your digestive health as well.

Let's start with yogurt—a classic probiotic food that many enjoy. Making yogurt at home is a straightforward process that requires little more than milk and a starter culture. Begin by heating your milk until it's just about to boil, then let it cool down to a temperature where it feels warm to the touch but not hot. Stir in a small amount of store-bought yogurt or starter culture, then transfer the mixture to a jar. Keep it in a warm place, like an oven with the light on, for about 8 to 12 hours. The result is a creamy, tangy yogurt rich in live cultures that enhance your gut flora. Enjoy it plain, or add a drizzle of honey and a handful of nuts for a satisfying breakfast or snack.

Sauerkraut is another gem in the world of fermentation. With just cabbage and salt, you can create a zesty, crunchy condiment that's teeming with probiotics. Start by shredding your cabbage finely and mixing it with salt in a large bowl. Knead and work the cabbage until it begins to release its juices. Pack it tightly into a glass jar, ensuring the cabbage is submerged in its liquid. Cover with a clean cloth and let it sit at room temperature for about a week, checking daily to ensure it stays submerged. The transformation is magical, as the cabbage ferments into a flavorful side dish that pairs beautifully with various meals.

Then, there are quick-pickled vegetables, which offer a toothsome punch and a probiotic boost. Choose your favorite vegetables—carrots, cucumbers, or radishes work well—and slice them thinly. Combine vinegar, water, salt, and a touch of sugar in a jar. Add your vegetables and any desired spices, such as dill or garlic. Let them marinate in the fridge for at least 24 hours. These pickles make a refreshing snack or a vibrant addition to sandwiches and salads, offering a burst of flavor and probiotics with every bite.

For breakfast, overnight oats with chia seeds and berries provide a nourishing start to the day. Simply combine rolled oats, chia seeds, and your choice of milk in a jar. Add a handful of berries for natural sweetness and a sprinkle of cinnamon for warmth. Let it sit in the fridge overnight. By morning, you'll have a creamy, fiber-rich breakfast that supports digestion and keeps you full and energized. This recipe is versatile—you can switch up the fruits or add a dollop of yogurt for an extra probiotic punch. Nothing could be easier!

Probiotic foods introduce beneficial bacteria into your gut, helping to balance the microbiome and support digestion. These bacteria aid in breaking down food and enhancing nutrient absorption, which can lead to improved energy levels and overall well-being. The beauty of these recipes lies not only in their simplicity but also in their adaptability. You can customize them to suit your preferences, adding spices or sweeteners for additional flavor. Add a refreshing twist to your yogurt with fresh herbs like mint or basil, or get creative with pickling by experimenting with different vegetables to uncover new flavor combinations.

REFLECTION SECTION

Consider how these recipes might fit into your lifestyle. Which ones intrigue you the most? Try one this week and observe how your body responds. Jot down any changes you notice in a journal, from energy levels to digestion. Engaging with your food in this way can deepen your appreciation for its healing potential.

SUPERFOOD SMOOTHIES AND INFUSIONS

When life gets hectic, as it often does, smoothies and infusions become my go-to for a quick, nutritious boost. Think of them as liquid gold for your gut, providing a concentrated source of vitamins, minerals, and gut-friendly ingredients in just a few sips. They're perfect for those mornings when you're rushing out the door or need a mid-afternoon pick-me-up. The beauty of smoothies lies in their convenience and versatility. You toss a variety of ingredients into a blender, and in moments, you have a vibrant, delicious drink. Infusions, on the other hand, offer a hydrating way to consume nutrients, perfect for when you want something lighter but still nourishing.

Consider starting your day with a green smoothie made with spinach, avocado, and kefir. The spinach provides a hefty dose of fiber and iron, while the avocado adds creaminess and healthy fats.

Kefir, a fermented milk drink, introduces beneficial probiotics to support your gut health. Blend these with a splash of water or coconut milk and perhaps a squeeze of lime for zest. The result is a refreshing beverage that fuels your day with sustained energy. For a sweeter option, try a berry and flaxseed smoothie. Berries like blueberries and strawberries are high in antioxidants, which combat oxidative stress, and flaxseeds add a nutty flavor with a dose of omega-3 fatty acids. Blend them with some almond milk and a touch of honey or maple syrup for sweetness, and you've got a fiber-rich treat that's as delicious as it's good for your gut. I always keep frozen bananas on hand to add to my smoothies—they enhance the texture and add variety to my breakfast options.

Infusions are another fantastic way to incorporate superfoods into your routine. Adding sliced cucumber, crushed mint, or berries can enhance water's flavor, making it more refreshing and enjoyable to drink. Consider a turmeric and ginger infusion. Turmeric is well-known for its anti-inflammatory properties; ginger adds warmth and aids digestion. Steep slices of fresh ginger and a teaspoon of ground turmeric in boiling water to make this infusion. Let it sit for a few minutes, then strain and enjoy. You can add a bit of honey if you like it sweeter. This soothing drink supports digestion and provides a calming start or end to your day.

Incorporating prebiotics and probiotics into these beverages can further enhance their gut health benefits. Prebiotics, which are non-digestible fibers, serve as food for the good bacteria in your gut. Try adding a spoonful of prebiotic fiber supplements, like inulin, to your smoothies. Probiotic powders or liquids can also be mixed into your drinks, adding a probiotic punch to boost your microbiome. These additions work synergistically to create a balanced environment in your gut, promoting digestion and overall wellness.

Creating balanced smoothies is all about combining ingredients that offer a variety of nutrients. Aim for a balance of macronutrients—

carbohydrates, proteins, and fats—to keep you energized and satisfied. For example, the carbohydrates in fruits offer a quick energy boost, while the healthy fats in avocados or nuts help maintain it. Adjust the sweetness with natural sweeteners, like honey or dates, considering your taste preferences and dietary needs. You can also experiment with different greens, seeds, or spices to find combinations you love.

Making smoothies and infusions is an opportunity to be creative. As you experiment, you'll find your favorite combinations that taste and make you feel great. They're a testament to the idea that caring for your gut doesn't have to be complicated or time-consuming, and it certainly isn't boring. It can be as simple as blending a few ingredients and sipping your way to better health. So grab your blender, gather some fresh ingredients, and see what delicious concoctions you can create. Your gut will thank you for it.

SNACKS AND DESSERTS - GUT-FRIENDLY TREATS

Who doesn't enjoy a delicious snack or sweet treat? They add little moments of joy to our daily routines but can sometimes feel like indulgences or guilty pleasures. The good news is that snacks and desserts can absolutely be part of a gut-friendly diet. It's all about making choices that satisfy cravings while supporting digestive health. Mindful indulgence is key. It's about savoring each bite with intention, choosing foods that nourish both your taste buds and gut. Imagine biting into something that tastes good and makes your body feel good. That's the magic of incorporating gut-supportive ingredients into your snacks and desserts.

Let's start with energy balls. These are perfect little bites made with oats, nuts, and dates. The oats provide fiber, the nuts offer healthy fats, and the dates add natural sweetness and essential minerals. To make these, blend a cup of rolled oats with a cup of mixed nuts—like almonds and walnuts—and a handful of pitted dates. Add a spoonful of chia seeds and a dash of cinnamon. Roll the mixture into balls and refrigerate them for a couple of hours. They're a quick, no-bake option that can be stored for days, making them perfect for a busy lifestyle. Each bite is a burst of energy, providing sustained fuel for your day.

Chia pudding is another delightful option. With a creamy texture and endless flavor possibilities, it's a versatile treat that satisfies your sweet tooth while nourishing your gut. Mix a quarter cup of chia seeds with one cup of coconut milk to prepare a basic chia pudding. Add a splash of vanilla extract and a tablespoon of maple syrup for sweetness. Stir well and let it sit in the fridge overnight. By morning, you'll have a thick, pudding-like consistency. Top with fresh berries, which are full of antioxidants, and add a sprinkle of nuts for added crunch. The chia seeds expand and soak up the liquid, creating a satisfying texture rich in omega-3 fatty acids.

Remember those frozen bananas you set aside for smoothies? Try blending a couple straight from the freezer, and you'll get a rich, nutty-flavored banana "ice cream" that's absolutely irresistible! Not only does it satisfy your ice cream cravings, it also serves as a delicious prebiotic treat to top off your meal.

If you love chocolate, dark chocolate bark with seeds and dried fruit could become your new go-to treat. Start by melting some good-quality dark chocolate. Spread it thinly on a lined baking sheet and sprinkle with sunflower seeds, pumpkin seeds, and your choice of dried fruits like cranberries or apricots. Set it in the fridge until firm, then break it into pieces. This bark is a perfect combination of sweet and savory, with the seeds adding fiber and healthy fats, while the dark chocolate provides antioxidants. It's a treat that feels indulgent but is packed with nutrients.

When choosing ingredients for these snacks and desserts, focus on natural sweeteners and whole ingredients. Honey, maple syrup, and stevia are excellent alternatives to refined sugar, providing sweetness without the blood sugar spikes. Whole grains like oats and nuts are nutrient-dense choices that support gut health. They add texture and flavor, and also enhance the nutritional profile of your treats. By making these mindful choices, you can enjoy snacks and desserts without compromising your digestive health.

Portion control and mindful eating are essential practices when enjoying these treats. It's easy to get carried away with delicious snacks, but moderation is key to maintaining gut health. Serve yourself a small portion, savor each bite, and listen to your body's hunger cues. Eating slowly and mindfully can enhance your enjoyment and prevent overeating. Focusing on the flavors and textures allows you to turn a simple snack into a moment of gratitude and self-care. Remember, it's not just about satisfying your cravings; it's about nourishing your body and treating yourself with kindness and respect.

MEAL PLANS FOR DIGESTIVE WELLNESS

Embracing the art of meal planning can transform how you approach your daily nutrition, especially when focusing on gut health. Meal planning isn't just about organization but ensuring your body consistently gets the diverse nutrients it craves. By planning your meals, you create a structured environment that supports your gut, helping it operate at its best. This reduces the stress of last-minute decisions and helps avoid the trap of convenient but less nutritious options.

Let's explore a sample meal plan to support your gut health throughout the day. Start with a breakfast of overnight oats with chia seeds. The oats provide a hearty base rich in fiber, while chia seeds offer omega-3s and a satisfying texture. Soak them overnight with your choice of milk and a sprinkle of cinnamon for added warmth. For lunch, a refreshing quinoa salad is both filling and gut-friendly. Toss cooked quinoa with mixed greens, fermented vegetables like kimchi or sauerkraut, and a drizzle of olive oil. The fermented veggies add tang and probiotics, enhancing the salad's nutritional profile. Dinner is a beautiful grilled salmon paired with roasted sweet potatoes. The salmon delivers essential omega-3 fatty acids, while sweet potatoes offer prebiotics and a touch of sweetness. For snacks throughout the day, keep it simple and satisfying with a handful of almonds and crunchy apple slices dipped in almond butter. These snacks are not only easy to prepare, they also sustain energy and aid digestion.

Meal planning doesn't mean rigid adherence to a set menu. Flexibility is crucial, especially when accommodating individual preferences and dietary restrictions. If you're dairy-free, swap out the milk in your oats for almond or coconut milk. Vegetarians might replace the salmon with a plant-based protein like lentils or chickpeas. Adjusting portion sizes is another way to tailor your meal plan. If you've had a particularly active day, increase your portions to meet your energy needs. Conversely, you might opt for lighter meals on a more sedentary day. This adaptability ensures that your meal plan remains a guide rather than a strict mandate.

Efficiency in meal prep can make the process smoother and more enjoyable. Consider setting aside time on the weekend for batch cooking. Prepare large quantities of grains, like quinoa or brown rice, and store them in the fridge for quick access. Roast various vegetables so you have a ready-to-eat lunch or dinner assortment. You can also get creative with leftovers. Turn last night's roasted vegetables into a hearty soup, or add them to a wrap for a different lunch experience. By organizing your prep time, you set yourself up for success, making it easier to stick to your gut-friendly plan even on the busiest of days.

This journey into meal planning is about cultivating a relationship with your food that honors your body's needs. As you explore these plans and adapt them to your life, you'll likely notice a shift in how you feel—more energy, better digestion, and perhaps a newfound appreciation for the vibrant foods that support your health. This chapter has touched on the influential role that meal planning has in digestive wellness, emphasizing the importance of structure, flexibility, and efficiency. As we move forward, the next chapter will explore the empowerment that comes with understanding and nurturing your digestive system, providing you with the knowledge and tools to continue shoring up your gut health on a daily basis.

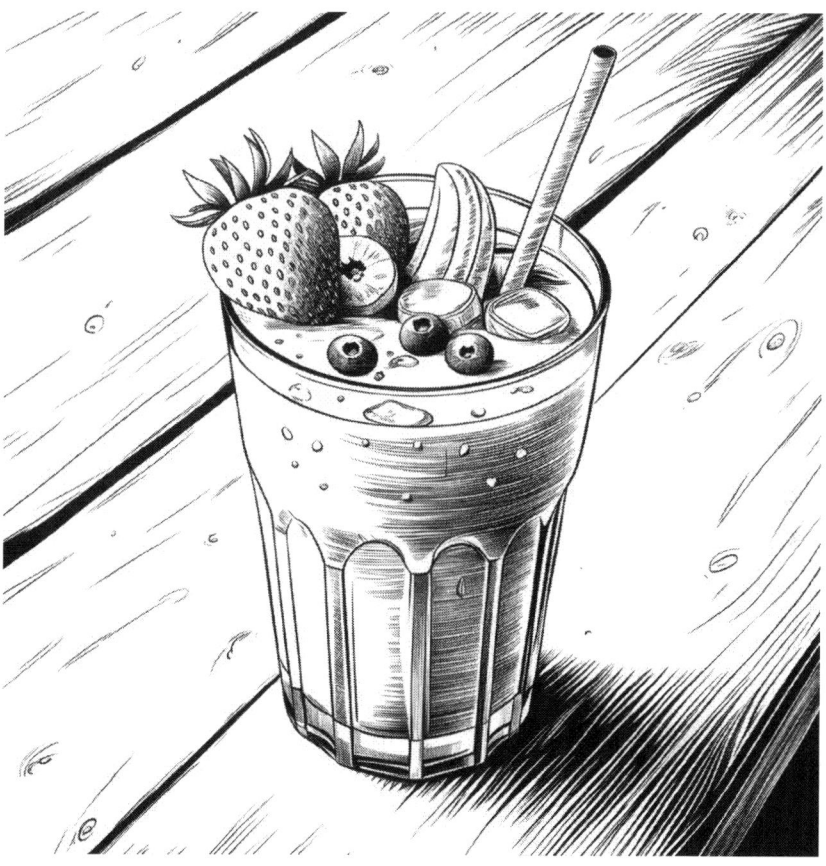

"Consistency is the key to success."

— UNKNOWN

12

EMPOWERMENT THROUGH KNOWLEDGE AND SELF-CARE

Picture yourself standing in front of a mirror—not just glancing but truly seeing yourself, noticing every detail that tells the story of your health journey. This is the heart of self-assessment—a powerful tool that reshapes how you understand and care for your gut health. It's about becoming your own health detective, deciphering the signals your body sends to identify patterns and triggers that influence your well-being. Regularly evaluating your digestive health is not just a routine task; it's an empowering practice that can lead to profound insights and proactive management of your health.

Self-assessment begins with awareness, and awareness starts with tracking. Keeping a symptom journal can be incredibly illuminating. It doesn't have to be complex—just a simple notebook or an app on your phone where you jot down what you eat and any digestive symptoms that follow. Over time, you'll notice patterns, like how certain foods may lead to discomfort or how stress affects your digestion. This increased awareness allows you to make connections that might otherwise go unnoticed, empowering you to make informed decisions about your diet and lifestyle.

Alongside a symptom journal, a food diary can be a valuable tool for identifying potential triggers. By chronicling your meals, snacks, and even beverages, you can pinpoint specific foods or combinations that might be causing issues. It's like creating a map of your digestive landscape, highlighting areas that need attention and adjustment. This process fosters a more in-depth understanding of how your body responds to different foods and encourages mindful eating as you become more intentional about what you consume.

For those who want to delve deeper, at-home testing kits can provide additional insights into your gut health. These kits, available online or through healthcare providers, can test for markers such as food sensitivities, microbial diversity, and even specific pathogens. While they don't replace professional medical advice, they can offer valuable information that complements your self-assessment efforts. Understanding these results can guide you in making targeted changes to your diet and lifestyle, helping you take proactive steps toward improving your gut health.

Once you've gathered your data, the next step is to interpret it. This means looking for trends and correlations between your diet, lifestyle, and symptoms. You may notice that dairy triggers bloating or that reducing sugar leads to clearer skin and better digestion. These observations are invaluable, as they highlight areas where you can make adjustments to improve your health. If you identify persistent issues or symptoms that don't resolve with dietary changes, it's important to consult a healthcare professional. They can provide further evaluation and develop a more comprehensive treatment plan.

Self-assessment is not just about identifying problems; it's about empowerment. You can tailor your health strategies to meet your unique needs with the information you've gathered. This might involve developing personalized dietary adjustments. It could also mean considering lifestyle changes, such as adopting stress-reduction techniques or adding regular exercise to your routine. By taking these steps, you're not just reacting to symptoms but actively shaping your health.

REFLECTION SECTION

As you embark on this self-assessment journey, consider setting aside a few minutes each day to reflect on your feelings and observations. Use this time to review your symptom journal and food diary, noting any patterns or changes. Ask yourself, "What foods made me feel good today?" or "What activities improved my digestion?" This reflective practice encourages a deeper connection with your body and fosters a sense of mindfulness in your daily life. It also offers a chance to celebrate small victories and track progress, reinforcing the positive changes you've made.

Self-assessment is a deeply personal process that invites you to listen closely to your body and trust in its wisdom. It's about embracing curiosity and compassion, and understanding that every piece of data you collect is a step toward greater health and well-being. By actively engaging in this practice, you empower yourself to make choices that support your unique needs, paving the way for a healthier, more vibrant life.

CREATING YOUR OWN GUT HEALTH PROTOCOL

Creating a personalized gut health protocol is like designing a custom suit that fits you perfectly, tailored to your unique lifestyle and needs. The first step is to set realistic and measurable objectives. Thinking about what you want to achieve can be as simple as reducing bloating or improving your energy levels. The key is to make these goals specific and attainable. You could start with a goal to include a daily serving of fermented foods or practice a stress-reducing activity twice a week. By setting clear targets, you give yourself a roadmap that guides your efforts toward tangible outcomes.

It's also essential to consider your genetic and cultural factors when developing your protocol. These aspects can significantly influence how your body responds to different foods and lifestyle changes. For example, certain genetic predispositions might make you more sensitive to specific dietary components, while cultural backgrounds can shape your eating habits and preferences. Embracing these factors allows you to craft a natural and sustainable protocol. This might mean incorporating traditional foods that resonate with your cultural heritage, providing comfort and familiarity while enhancing your gut health.

A well-rounded gut health protocol also includes lifestyle and stress management components. Recognizing the impact of stress on your digestive system is crucial, as it can worsen symptoms and disrupt your microbiome. Incorporating yoga, meditation, or even simple breathing exercises can help keep stress levels in check. Similarly, regular physical activity promotes digestion and overall well-being, making it important to find an exercise routine you enjoy as part of your protocol. Remember to celebrate the small victories along the way—each positive change, no matter how minor it may seem, is a step toward improved gut health.

While you can do much of this independently, integrating professional guidance ensures your protocol is balanced and safe. Consulting with nutritionists or gastroenterologists provides insights into your specific health needs. They can offer professional assessments and testing, such as comprehensive stool analysis or food sensitivity testing, to help identify underlying issues. With evidence-based recommendations from healthcare providers, you can refine your approach to address deficiencies or imbalances that might not be apparent through self-assessment alone.

Crafting your protocol is an opportunity for creativity and adaptation. For example, if increasing fiber and prebiotic intake is a priority, you might start by introducing more whole grains, fruits, and vegetables into your meals. Adding probiotic-rich foods like yogurt or kefir can enrich your diet. On the other hand, if stress reduction and exercise are more critical, you might focus on incorporating daily walks or joining a local yoga class. The beauty of a personalized plan is its ability to evolve with you, reflecting changes in your lifestyle, goals, and health status.

Flexibility is vital in maintaining an effective gut health plan. As you continue to evaluate your health, you may need to adjust your strategies in response to new insights or symptoms. You may notice that a particular food consistently triggers discomfort, prompting you to modify your dietary choices. You may also find that a new exercise routine enhances your digestive health, leading you to incorporate it more regularly. Periodic review and refinement of your approach ensures it stays aligned with your needs, promoting your well-being as you move forward.

Developing a gut health protocol is an empowering journey of self-discovery and care. It's about embracing your uniqueness, understanding what works best for you, and making intentional choices that benefit your health. By setting clear goals, seeking expert advice, and staying flexible, you can create a plan that boosts your gut health and enhances your life in meaningful ways.

LONG-TERM STRATEGIES FOR SUSTAINED WELL-BEING

In the rush of daily life, it's tempting to look for quick fixes, especially when it comes to our health. But here's a little secret: lasting wellness is rooted in sustainable habits. It's like tending to a garden—you can't simply water the seeds once and expect them to bloom overnight. It takes consistent care, attention, and patience. Likewise, when it comes to gut health, it's about nurturing habits that slowly transform our daily routines and create a lasting impact over time.

Start with small, achievable goals that align with your lifestyle. It may mean swapping out that mid-morning pastry for a piece of fruit or adding a short walk after dinner. These changes may seem minor, but they're stepping stones to more significant shifts. Setting specific objectives creates a sense of direction, much like mapping out a journey. Each goal reached is a victory worth celebrating, no matter how small it may seem. These milestones mark progress and reinforce your commitment, motivating you to continue on the path toward wellness.

Consistency is the glue that holds these habits together. It's about showing up for yourself day after day, even when motivation wanes. Think of it as a promise you make to your future self—an investment in your long-term health. When you commit to these practices, you build a solid foundation that supports your well-being amid life's inevitable ups and downs. This consistency turns new behaviors into second nature, making them an integral part of your lifestyle.

So, what does a sustainable approach to gut health look like? It starts with regular incorporation of fiber and fermented foods into your diet. Fiber is nature's broom, sweeping through your digestive system and promoting regularity. Meanwhile, fermented foods like yogurt, kimchi, and sauerkraut introduce beneficial bacteria that can enhance your gut flora. These foods don't just help with digestion; they nourish your body, providing the nutrients needed for energy and vitality. Making them a staple in your meals can have profound effects over time, supporting a healthy microbiome that thrives on diversity.

Equally important is maintaining regular physical activity and managing stress. Exercise doesn't have to mean hitting the gym every day. It can be as simple as a brisk walk, a dance class, or even playing with your kids in the park. The key is to find activities you enjoy, ensuring you stick with them. Exercise stimulates digestion and promotes mental clarity, contributing to overall wellness. Paired with stress management techniques—meditation, deep breathing, or simply taking time to unwind—exercise becomes a powerful tool in your health arsenal.

Mindfulness and self-care are at the heart of long-term wellness. Mindful eating, for example, encourages you to savor each bite, fostering a deeper connection with your food and enhancing digestion. This practice invites you to be present and attentive, reducing the likelihood of overeating and promoting satisfaction. Beyond the table, self-care routines prioritizing mental and emotional well-being are crucial. Whether journaling, taking a warm bath, or engaging in a creative hobby, self-care nurtures the soul, creating a balanced life that supports your entire being.

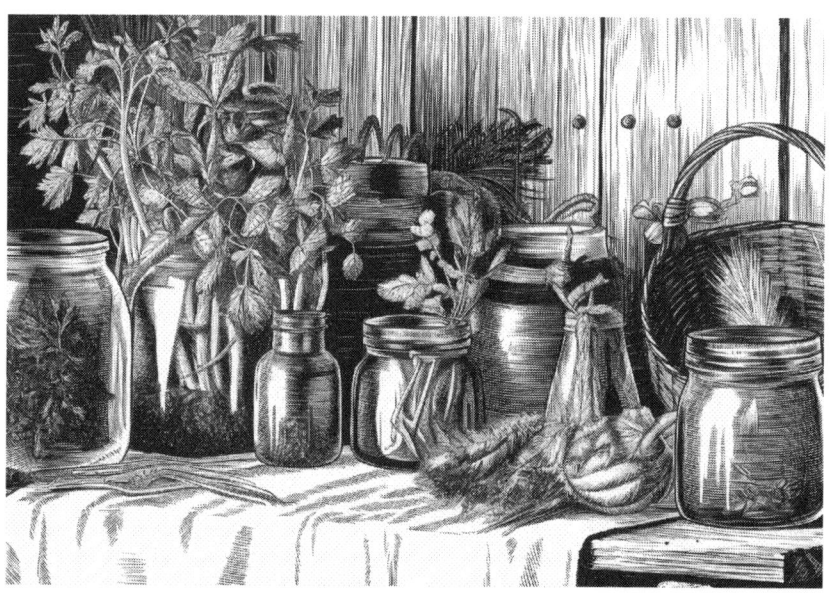

Taking charge of your health journey requires a proactive mindset. It's an invitation to engage with your well-being, making conscious choices that align with your values and goals. By remaining actively involved, you cultivate a sense of empowerment, knowing you hold the reins to your health. This engagement fuels motivation, inspiring you to explore new strategies, seek knowledge, and adapt as needed.

As we transition into the next chapter, let's remember that each step, no matter how small, contributes to the bigger picture of our health. It's a continuous process that evolves with us as we grow and change. The journey may not always be linear, but with commitment and care, the rewards are well worth the effort.

13
YOUR DIGESTIVE SYSTEM - AN OVERVIEW

The digestive system is one of the most complex systems in the body, responsible for breaking down food, absorbing nutrients, and eliminating waste. In this chapter, we'll explore the key organs of digestion, as well as common digestive issues. We will conclude with a glossary of key terms to enhance your understanding of the digestive system and its processes, empowering you to make informed choices for long-term wellness.

KEY DIGESTIVE ORGANS

Your digestive system is like an assembly line, where each organ contributes to breaking down food into nutrients your body needs. The stomach acts like a powerful blender and chemical reactor. Once you chew and swallow your food, the stomach's muscular walls churn and mix it with gastric juices—composed of hydrochloric acid and enzymes like pepsin. This acidic environment is crucial; it breaks down proteins into smaller chains of amino acids and kills harmful bacteria that might have hitched a ride with your meal. The stomach's role is not just to pulverize food mechanically but also to prepare it chemically for the next stage of digestion.

The nutrient-rich chyme, which is what food becomes after its time in the stomach, makes its way into the small intestine. This long, coiled tube is where most of the magic happens, and its primary task is nutrient absorption. The small intestine's lining is covered with tiny, finger-like projections called villi, which increase the surface area for absorption. Here, enzymes from the pancreas and bile from the liver further break down carbohydrates, proteins, and fats into their simplest forms: sugars, amino acids, and fatty acids. These nutrients are absorbed through the villi and into the bloodstream, transporting them to cells throughout the body. The small intestine is not just a passive player; it actively selects and absorbs the nutrients your body needs, ensuring that every meal you eat contributes to your energy levels and overall health.

As food moves through the digestive tract, it eventually reaches the large intestine or colon. The colon's primary function is to absorb water and electrolytes from the remaining indigestible food matter, transforming it from a liquid mush into solid stool. Picture the colon as a recycling plant, where water is reclaimed and waste is compacted for expulsion. This process helps maintain your body's hydration levels and is crucial in detoxification. As the colon absorbs water, it ferments any remaining carbohydrates with the help of your gut flora, producing short-chain fatty acids that provide additional energy and aid in maintaining a healthy microbiome. The colon's rhythm, known as peristalsis, ensures that waste is moved efficiently toward the rectum, where it's stored until you're ready to eliminate it.

Understanding the roles these key digestive organs play can empower you to make dietary and lifestyle choices that support their function. Whether it's the stomach's role in kick-starting digestion, the small intestine's nutrient absorption, or the colon's water reclamation, each organ plays a vital part in maintaining the balance and health of your digestive system. By appreciating how these components work in harmony, you gain insight into the importance of nurturing your digestive health.

COMMON DIGESTIVE DISORDERS - A SUMMARY

- **Celiac disease:** an autoimmune disorder where consuming gluten triggers an immune response that damages the small intestine lining. This damage impairs nutrient absorption and can cause symptoms like diarrhea, bloating, fatigue, and weight loss. Long-term effects can include malnutrition and other complications. The only treatment is a strict, lifelong gluten-free diet.
- **Crohn's disease:** a chronic inflammatory bowel disease (IBD) that causes inflammation in the digestive tract, most commonly affecting the small intestine and colon. Symptoms include abdominal pain, diarrhea, weight loss, and fatigue. The exact cause is unknown, but is thought to involve an immune system malfunction. Treatment often includes medication to control inflammation, and in some cases, surgery.
- **Irritable Bowel Syndrome (IBS):** a common and complex condition causing symptoms like bloating, gas, abdominal pain, constipation, diarrhea, or a mix of both. Its cause remains unclear but is linked to stress, diet, and gut sensitivity. It doesn't cause intestinal damage but significantly impacts quality of life.
- **Gluten intolerance:** a condition where the body reacts negatively to gluten, a protein found in wheat, barley, and rye. Symptoms can include bloating, gas, diarrhea, fatigue, and headaches. While it doesn't cause long-term damage to the intestines, it can significantly affect digestion and

overall well-being. Managing gluten intolerance typically involves following a gluten-free diet.
- **Lactose intolerance:** the inability to properly digest lactose, the sugar found in milk and dairy products, due to a deficiency in lactase, the enzyme needed for digestion. This can lead to symptoms like bloating, diarrhea, and stomach cramps after consuming dairy. It can often be managed by reducing or eliminating dairy intake or using lactase supplements.
- **Leaky Gut Syndrome:** not officially recognized as a medical condition, it involves increased intestinal permeability, where the gut lining becomes too porous, allowing harmful particles to pass into the bloodstream. This can cause digestive symptoms and other health issues like fatigue and joint pain. More research is needed to confirm its effects and implications.
- **Small Intestinal Bacterial Overgrowth (SIBO):** occurs when there's an abnormal increase in bacteria in the small intestine. It leads to symptoms similar to IBS—bloating, gas, and discomfort—and can cause nutrient malabsorption. Factors like altered gut motility and surgery complications may trigger it. Treatment often involves diet changes, antibiotics, and sometimes probiotics.
- **Small Intestinal Fungal Overgrowth (SIFO):** happens when excessive fungal growth, often candida, occurs in the small intestine. It can cause symptoms like bloating, gas, and abdominal discomfort, and may lead to nutrient malabsorption. Contributing factors include antibiotic use, a weakened immune system, and gut imbalances. Treatment typically involves antifungal medications and dietary changes.

Bloating, gas, and abdominal pain are common symptoms across many of these disorders. Their presence can cause discomfort and concern, as well as confusion, since they appear in most of these conditions. Bloating is that uncomfortable swelling sensation in the abdomen, often accompanied by visible distention. It's usually caused by excess gas production or disturbances in the movement of the digestive tract muscles. Gas, a normal part of digestion, can be problematic when excessive or trapped, leading to pain and embarrassment. Abdominal pain, which can vary in intensity and location, often signals that something isn't quite right. Paying attention to these symptoms is crucial, as they can indicate underlying digestive issues that might need addressing.

Understanding these disorders is not just about identifying symptoms, but also about recognizing their impact on daily life. Many people with these conditions face challenges that extend beyond the physical discomfort, affecting their social interactions, mental health, and overall well-being. It's essential to approach these issues with empathy and an open mind, seeking support and professional guidance when needed. Acknowledging the reality of these disorders can be the first step towards finding effective management strategies and improving one's quality of life.

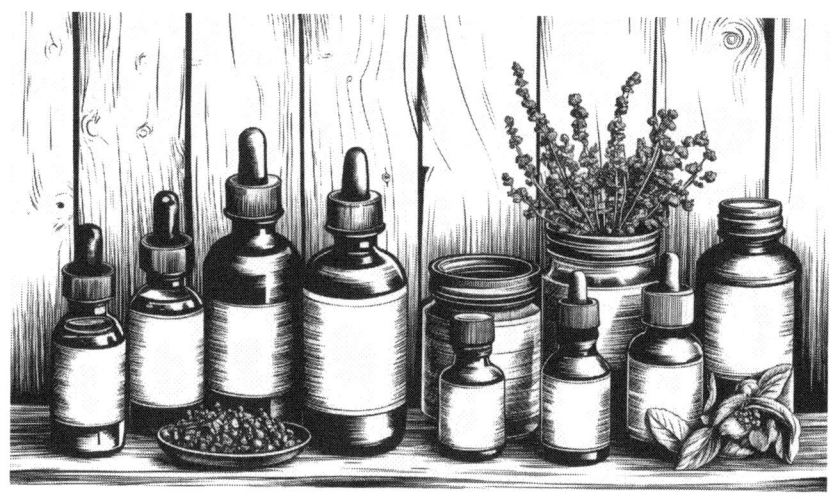

"The journey is the reward."

— CHINESE PROVERB

GLOSSARY OF TERMS

From the moment you take a bite of food, various processes begin that transform the food into the energy and nutrients your body needs. This section will help you understand this complex system by introducing a glossary of terms. Defining these terms can demystify the digestive process and clarify how our bodies work.

Acetate - a short-chain fatty acid (SCFA) produced during the fermentation of dietary fibers by gut bacteria in the colon, that plays a vital role in gut health by helping to maintain the integrity of the intestinal lining, supporting the growth of beneficial gut bacteria, and providing energy to colon cells. It is also absorbed into the bloodstream and can have systemic effects on metabolism and inflammation.

Adenosine Triphosphate (ATP) - a molecule that serves as the primary source of energy for most cellular processes in the body.

Allium - plants known for their distinctive aromas and flavors, such as garlic, onions, leeks, shallots, and chives, often used to enhance the taste of dishes, and valued for their potential health benefits.

GLOSSARY OF TERMS

Anaerobic - conditions or organisms that do not require oxygen to live or grow.

Antimicrobial - a substance that kills or inhibits the growth of microorganisms, such as bacteria, fungi, viruses, or parasites.

Antinutrients - naturally occurring compounds found in many plant-based foods that can interfere with the absorption of nutrients or have other negative effects on health.

Autoimmune - a condition in which the body's immune system mistakenly attacks its own healthy cells, tissues, or organs, leading to inflammation and damage.

Beta-glucan - a type of soluble fiber found in the cell walls of certain grains (like oats and barley), fungi (such as yeast and mushrooms), and some bacteria. It is known for its potential health benefits, particularly for heart health and immune system support and has been studied for its potential to support digestive health and improve blood sugar regulation.

Butyrate - a short-chain fatty acid (SCFA) produced by the fermentation of dietary fibers by gut bacteria, particularly in the colon. It's an important fuel source for the cells lining the gut and plays a critical role in maintaining gut health by promoting the integrity of the intestinal barrier. It also has anti-inflammatory properties and regulates immune function.

Cardiometabolic - interrelated factors that influence the risk of both cardiovascular diseases (such as heart disease and stroke) and metabolic conditions (such as type 2 diabetes, obesity, and metabolic syndrome).

Carminative - substances, typically herbs or plants, that help relieve gas, bloating, and discomfort in the digestive system.

Chyme - the partially digested, semi-liquid food mixture that forms in the stomach after food is broken down by mechanical and chemical processes.

Circadian - biological processes or rhythms that follow a roughly 24-hour cycle, responding to external cues such as light and darkness, affecting various functions in the body, including sleep-wake cycles, hormone release, and metabolism.

Coenzymes - small organic molecules that assist enzymes in catalyzing biochemical reactions. Many coenzymes are derived from vitamins or other essential nutrients.

Cognitive Behavioral Therapy (CBT) - a type of psychotherapy that focuses on identifying and changing negative thought patterns and behaviors that contribute to emotional distress and mental health issues. CBT is based on the idea that our thoughts, feelings, and behaviors are interconnected, and by changing negative thought patterns, we can improve emotional well-being and develop healthier behaviors.

Cortisol - plays a crucial role in regulating various body functions, including metabolism, immune response, and inflammation. It helps the body respond to stress by increasing blood sugar levels, enhancing the brain's use of glucose, and providing energy for the "fight or flight" response.

Crohn's Disease - a chronic inflammatory bowel disease (IBD) that causes inflammation, irritation, and swelling of the digestive tract, most commonly affecting the small intestine and colon.

Cruciferous - a family of vegetables including a variety of nutrient-dense, leafy greens such as broccoli, cauliflower, kale, Brussels sprouts, cabbage, and bok choy that are rich in fiber, vitamins, minerals, and phytochemicals, and linked to supporting digestive and immune health.

GLOSSARY OF TERMS

Deglycyrrhizinated - a process in which glycyrrhizin, the active compound in licorice root, is removed or reduced to make the product safer for use, particularly for individuals with high blood pressure or those sensitive to its effects.

Disaccharides - a type of carbohydrate made up of two simple sugar molecules such as sucrose (table sugar), lactose (the sugar found in milk), and maltose (found in malted foods and beer).

Dopamine - a chemical messenger in the brain that plays a key role in mood regulation, motivation, reward, pleasure, and motor control.

Dysbiosis - an imbalance or disruption in the normal composition of the microbiota, particularly the gut microbiome, where harmful microorganisms (like pathogenic bacteria or fungi) outnumber beneficial ones leading to various health issues, such as digestive problems, inflammation, autoimmune conditions, and even mood disorders.

Electrolytes - minerals that carry an electric charge when dissolved in water. They are essential for a variety of bodily functions, including maintaining fluid balance, regulating muscle and nerve function, and supporting proper hydration.

Endorphins - natural chemicals produced by the brain and nervous system that act as neurotransmitters, helping to relieve pain and reduce stress. Often referred to as the body's "feel-good" hormones, endorphins promote feelings of euphoria, happiness, and well-being.

Gamma-aminobutyric acid (GABA) - a neurotransmitter in the brain that plays a key role in helping to calm the nervous system by inhibiting overactive brain activity. This function is essential for promoting relaxation, reducing stress, and preventing excessive stimulation in the brain, and is involved in regulating muscle tone, mood, and sleep.

Ghrelin - a hormone primarily produced by the stomach that plays a key role in regulating hunger and appetite.

Glucose - a simple sugar and primary source of energy for the body's cells, it is absorbed into the bloodstream after the digestion of carbohydrates.

Gluten - a group of proteins found in grains such as wheat, barley, and rye. It gives dough its elasticity and helps baked goods maintain their shape and chewy texture.

Glycyrrhizin - a natural compound found in licorice root that is responsible for the sweet flavor of licorice. It has been used in traditional medicine for its potential health benefits, including its anti-inflammatory, antiviral, and immune-boosting properties. However, it can have side effects, such as raising blood pressure, reducing potassium levels, and causing water retention, especially when consumed in large amounts.

Gut-brain axis - the bidirectional communication network between the gut and the brain, involving neural, hormonal, and immune pathways. This connection allows the gut and brain to influence each other's functions, affecting digestion, mood, cognition, and overall health.

Gut flora - refers to the trillions of microorganisms (such as bacteria, viruses, fungi, and other microbes) that live in the digestive system, primarily in the intestines. These microbes play a crucial role in digestion, immunity, and overall health, breaking down food, producing vitamins, regulating the immune system, and protecting against harmful pathogens.

Immunoglobulins - proteins produced by the immune system to help identify and neutralize harmful substances like bacteria, viruses, and toxins.

GLOSSARY OF TERMS

Insulin - a hormone produced by the pancreas that plays a crucial role in regulating blood sugar (glucose) levels.

Inulin - a type of prebiotic fiber found in many plants that supports gut health by feeding beneficial bacteria in the intestines.

L-glutamine - a naturally occurring amino acid that plays a crucial role in various bodily functions, including gut health, immune support, and muscle recovery. It can also be found as a supplement.

Lactase - an enzyme produced in the small intestine that is responsible for breaking down lactose, the sugar found in milk and dairy products.

Lactose - a type of sugar found naturally in milk and dairy products.

Lactulos-Mannitol - a diagnostic test used to assess intestinal permeability, often referred to as leaky gut syndrome. It measures how well the lining of the intestines is functioning by analyzing the absorption of these two sugar molecules.

Leptin - a hormone primarily produced by fat cells that helps regulate appetite and energy balance by signaling to the brain when the body has enough stored fat.

Maltose - also known as "malt sugar", it is commonly found in foods like malted grains, as well as in the process of starch digestion, particularly carbohydrates.

Melatonin - a hormone that is primarily produced by the pineal gland in the brain, especially in response to darkness. It regulates the body's sleep-wake cycle.

Microbiome - consists of trillions of microorganisms, including bacteria, viruses, fungi, and other microbes, that live in your digestive tract. These tiny creatures play vital roles in digestion and immunity, and even impact your mood and mental health.

GLOSSARY OF TERMS

Microbiota - refers to the collection of microorganisms, such as bacteria, viruses, fungi, and other microbes, that inhabit a specific environment in the body.

Monosaccharides - "simple sugars" that are easily absorbed by the body and rapidly utilized for energy. They can be absorbed directly into the bloodstream through the intestines without needing to be broken down further.

Motility - movements of the digestive tract that help propel food and waste through the system.

Neurotransmitters - chemical messengers that transmit signals between nerve cells (neurons) in the brain and throughout the nervous system. They play a key role in communication within the brain, influencing mood, behavior, movement, and various bodily functions.

Oligosaccharides - a type of carbohydrate found in a variety of foods, including beans, vegetables, and whole grains, acting as a source of energy and playing a role in gut health.

Omega-3 Fatty Acids - a group of polyunsaturated fats essential for human health that the body cannot produce on its own, so they must be obtained through diet or supplements. Omega-3 fatty acids play important roles in brain function, inflammation reduction, and heart health.

Parasympathetic - one of the two main branches of the autonomic nervous system, responsible for promoting a state of relaxation and recovery after stress.

Pathogens - microorganisms, such as bacteria, viruses, fungi, or parasites, that cause disease or infection in a host organism.

Pepsin - an enzyme found in the stomach that plays a crucial role in the digestion of proteins.

GLOSSARY OF TERMS

Peptide YY - a hormone produced primarily in the intestines in response to food intake. It plays a key role in regulating appetite and energy balance.

Peristalsis - describes the wave-like muscle contractions that move food through your gastrointestinal tract from the esophagus, stomach, small intestine, and into the large intestine.

Phytonutrients - naturally occurring compounds found in plants that benefit human health, support overall health, and help prevent chronic diseases.

Polyols - used as sweeteners and bulking agents in a variety of food products, especially those marketed as "sugar-free" or "low-calorie." They occur naturally in some fruits and vegetables, but they are also synthetically produced for use in food and beverages.

Polysaccharides - complex carbohydrates, made up of hundreds or thousands of sugar molecules found in foods like potatoes, rice, and corn.

Prebiotics - non-digestible fibers found in foods such as fruits, vegetables, legumes, and whole grains. They serve as food for probiotics, helping them grow and function effectively.

Probiotics - friendly bacteria living in your gut that can be supplemented through certain foods or pills. They help maintain the balance of your gut microbiome, supporting digestion and boosting your immune system, as well as warding off harmful bacteria and creating a healthy environment. Probiotic supplements vary in quality and strain specificity, so choosing the right one can make a difference.

Propionate - a type of short-chain fatty acid (SCFA) that is produced in the gut during the fermentation of dietary fiber, particularly from foods such as whole grains, vegetables, and legumes. It helps maintain the gut microbiome's balance, supports the intestinal lining's health, and can reduce inflammation. It is also thought to have potential benefits for managing blood sugar levels and reducing the risk of metabolic diseases.

Reiki - a form of alternative therapy that involves channeling energy through a practitioner's hands to promote healing and balance in the recipient's body, mind, and spirit. The practice is based on the belief that there is a universal life force energy that flows through all living things and that this energy can be harnessed to promote physical, emotional, and spiritual well-being.

Serotonin - a neurotransmitter that plays a crucial role in regulating various bodily functions and is often referred to as the "feel-good" chemical due to its influence on mood, emotions, and overall sense of well-being.

Sucrose - commonly known as table sugar and is widely used as a sweetener in food and beverages.

Symbiotic - a mutually beneficial relationship between two different organisms living in close association.

Sympathetic - one part of the autonomic nervous system, which controls involuntary functions in the body. It is often referred to as the "fight or flight" system because it is activated during stressful or threatening situations, preparing the body to respond to danger.

Synergistic - the concept of two or more elements working together in a way that produces a combined effect greater than the sum of their individual effects.

Vagus nerve - part of the parasympathetic nervous system, which is responsible for regulating functions that occur automatically, such as heart rate, digestion, and respiratory rate. The vagus nerve is involved in the gut-brain axis, a bidirectional communication pathway between the gut and the brain and helps transmit signals related to gut health, hunger, and satiety.

GLOSSARY OF TERMS

Villi - tiny, finger-like projections in the small intestine that absorb nutrients and ensure your body receives the essential vitamins, minerals, proteins, and fats needed for energy, growth, and cell repair.

Understanding these terms and processes can empower you to make informed decisions about your digestive health. By appreciating how your body works, you can better support it through diet, lifestyle, and mindful choices. Remember, your digestive system is a remarkable network that deserves care and attention, much like a well-tuned machine that keeps you moving through life with energy and vitality.

As we wrap up this chapter, it's evident that understanding the digestive system is about recognizing the bigger picture—how our bodies convert food into the vital fuel we need to thrive. The interconnectedness of each organ and process highlights the importance of maintaining digestive health for overall well-being.

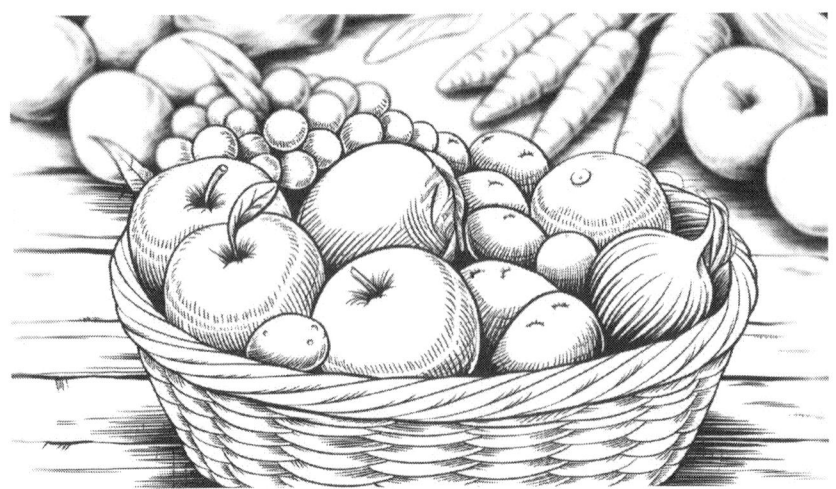

CONCLUSION

As we end our journey through the fascinating world of gut health, I want to reflect on the incredible insights and discoveries we've made together. By sharing my story and the wealth of knowledge I've gathered, I hope I've inspired you to take charge of your gut health and embrace the power of natural healing.

Throughout these pages, we've explored the intricate connection between our digestive system and overall well-being. From the benefits of fiber and fermented foods to the importance of stress management and mindful eating, we've uncovered a treasure trove of strategies to support our digestive health.

True wellness is not about perfection or quick fixes. It's about the small, consistent choices we make every day—the foods we eat, how we move our bodies, and the thoughts we choose to focus on. It's about listening to our gut, both literally and figuratively, and honoring its wisdom. And it's about embracing the journey, with all its ups and downs, knowing that each step brings us closer to a healthier, more vibrant version of ourselves.

CONCLUSION

So, as you close this book, remember that you have the power to transform your digestive health, one small change at a time. Embrace the magic of fermented foods, the nourishment of whole, plant-based ingredients, and the joy of mindful eating. Cultivate a sense of wonder and appreciation for the incredible work your body does every day to keep you healthy and energized.

Most importantly, trust in yourself and the innate wisdom of your gut. Listen to its signals, honor its needs, and treat it with the kindness and respect it deserves. When you do, you'll discover a level of well-being that radiates from the inside out, infusing every aspect of your life with vitality and joy.

Thank you for joining me on this incredible journey. Here's to your health, happiness, and the incredible power of a thriving gut!

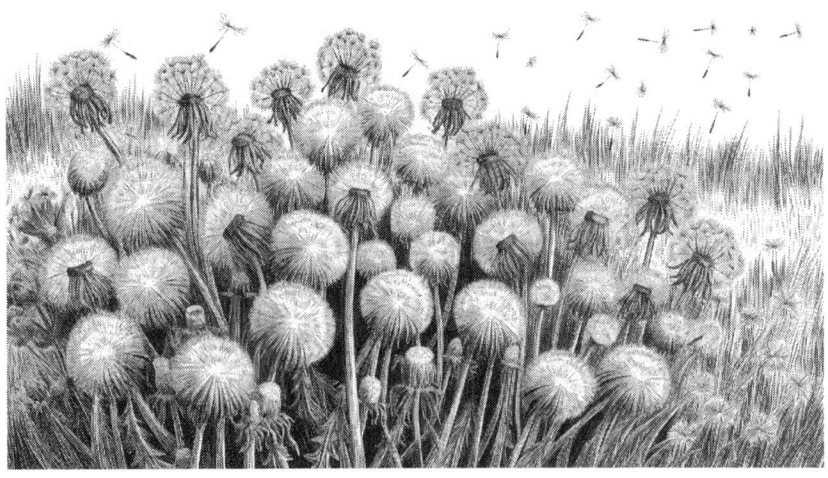

SHARE THE JOURNEY

As you turn the last page of this book, I hope you're feeling empowered—like you finally have the tools to nourish your gut, restore balance, and take charge of your health. Maybe you've already noticed small changes—a calmer stomach, steadier energy, or just the relief of knowing you're on the right path.

Now, it's your turn to help someone else.

Most of us find books through the words of others. By sharing your honest thoughts on Amazon, you can guide fellow readers who are searching for the same answers you once were. Your review might be the reason someone takes that first step toward healing.

Thank you for being part of this journey. *The Gut Health Solution* lives on when we pass our knowledge forward—and you're helping to do just that.

https://www.amazon.com/review/review-your-purchases/?asin=B0FC6X53CM

Act as if what you do makes a difference. It does."

— WILLIAM JAMES

BIBLIOGRAPHY

- AAJJO. (n.d.). *ACV gummies: Benefits of apple cider vinegar gummies for digestive health.* https://blog.aajjo.com/post/benefits-of-apple-cider-vinegar-gummies-for-digestive-health
- Acaria Health. (n.d.). *Understanding the role of the colon in chronic diarrhea.* https://acariahealth-envolvehealth.su/understanding-the-role-of-the-colon-in-chronic-diarrhea
- Advanced Food Intolerance Labs. (n.d.). *Identifying trigger foods: A guide for those with digestive issues and food intolerances.* Advanced Food Intolerance Labs. https://advancedfoodintolerancelabs.com/blogs/news/identifying-trigger-foods-a-guide-for-those-with-digestive-issues-and-food-intolerances
- Agape Nutrition. (n.d.). *SIBO: What is it? Small intestinal bacterial overgrowth.* https://agapenutrition.com/blogs/videos/sibo-what-is-it-small-intestinal-bacterial-overgrowth
- Albrecht, L., & McCaw, J. (2017). Using QR codes to connect patients to health information. *Journal of Medical Internet Research, 19*(8), e284. https://doi.org/10.2196/jmir.7366
- All Recipes. (n.d.). *Prebiotic and probiotic recipes.* All Recipes. Retrieved February 2, 2025, from https://www.allrecipes.com/recipes/17625/healthy-recipes/prebiotic-and-probiotic/
- America's Clinic. (2023, October 17). *The gut-brain connection: Probiotics, mental health, and overall well-being.* America's Clinic. https://americasclinic.com/blog/the-gut-brain-connection
- American College of Gastroenterology. (n.d.). *Irritable bowel syndrome (IBS) screener.* American College of Gastroenterology. Retrieved February 2, 2025, from https://gi.org/patients/ibs-screener/
- Atlas Bar. (n.d.). *What is the carnivore diet? A comprehensive guide.* https://atlasbars.com/blogs/nutrition-glossary/what-is-the-carnivore-diet-a-comprehensive-guide
- Author(s). (2024). Antibiotics and the gut microbiome: Understanding the impact. *Journal Name, Volume*(Issue), Page numbers. https://www.sciencedirect.com/science/article/pii/S2590097824000090
- Author(s). (Year). Dietary fiber intake and gut microbiota in human health. *PubMed Central.* https://pmc.ncbi.nlm.nih.gov/articles/PMC9787832/

BIBLIOGRAPHY

- Bastos, L. M., Pimentel, G. M., Costa, L. A., & Silva, C. A. (2022). Gut-brain axis: Investigating the effects of gut microbiota on neurodevelopment and neurological diseases. *Journal of Neuroinflammation, 19*(1), 75. https://doi.org/10.1186/s12974-022-02329-2
- Belkaid, Y., & Hand, T. W. (2014). Role of the normal gut microbiota. *Immunity, 42*(3), 1–12. https://doi.org/10.1016/j.immuni.2014.09.008
- Belmar Pharma Solutions. (n.d.). *Foundations of gut health*. Belmar Pharma Solutions. https://www.belmarpharmasolutions.com/resources/clinician-resources/clinician-library/foundations-of-gut-health/
- Berkheiser, K. (2019, March 27). *6 emerging benefits and uses of carom seeds (Ajwain)*. Healthline. https://www.healthline.com/nutrition/carom-seeds
- Bimuno. (2024, February 2). *5 apps for IBS and digestive health in 2024*. Retrieved February 2, 2025, from https://www.bimuno.com/news/gut-health/5-apps-for-ibs-and-digestive-health-in-2024/?srsltid=AfmBOooB3giCIV3fCbICRoNn_jUt3g-daFeVdQJYMgK-sAUzdxfWR37I
- Biosphere Nutrition. (n.d.). *The impact of prebiotics on gut health and autoimmune conditions*. Biosphere Nutrition. https://www.biospherenutrition.co.nz/blogs/prebiotics/the-impact-of-prebiotics-on-gut-health-and-autoimmune-conditions
- Bulletin 1247. (2024, April). *The journey of food through the human body!* https://www.bulletin1247.com.ng/2024/04/the-journey-of-food-through-human-body.html
- Butler, N. (2023, August 10). *Support your magical microbiome from top to toe: Gut, skin, mouth & intimate areas*. Biobod. https://www.biobod.com.au/blogs/news/support-your-magical-microbiome
- Calm Egg. (2023, July 1). *9 best strategies for anxiety relief through meditation*. Calm Egg. https://calmegg.com/mindful-meditation-for-anxiety-relief/
- Cani, P. D., & Everard, A. (2013). Effects of gut microbes on nutrient absorption and energy regulation. *Current Opinion in Clinical Nutrition & Metabolic Care, 16*(4), 409-414. https://doi.org/10.1097/MCO.0b013e3283603722
- Casa de Sante. (n.d.). *Casa de Sante's approach to prebiotics and your microbiome*. Casa de Sante. https://casadesante.com/blogs/gut-health/casa-de-sante-s-approach-to-prebiotics-and-your-microbiome
- Casa de Sante. (n.d.). *Complete food sensitivity profile: 210 foods IgA & IgG by Vibrant Wellness vs. blood typing*. Casa de Sante. https://casadesante.com/blogs/food-sensitivity-tests/complete-food-sensitivity-profile-210-foods-iga-igg-by-vibrant-wellness-vs-blood-typing
- CentreSpringMD. (n.d.). *Building a healthy gut: The 5R protocol and functional medicine testing*. CentreSpringMD. Retrieved February 2, 2025,

- from https://centrespringmd.com/building-a-healthy-gut-the-5r-protocol-and-functional-medicine-testing/?srsltid=AfmBOorriyneFz YKz2JJgyHgbGA-GLtEE0hylDazj2tN16dKaKKyCZEb
- Cleveland Clinic. (2022, July 14). *How exercise can lead to a healthy gut.* Cleveland Clinic. https://health.clevelandclinic.org/gut-health-workout
- Cleveland Clinic. (n.d.). *Leaky gut syndrome: Symptoms, diet, tests & treatment.* https://my.clevelandclinic.org/health/diseases/22724-leaky-gut-syndrome
- Complement. (n.d.). *Personalized nutrition quiz.* Complement. Retrieved February 2, 2025, from https://lovecomplement.com/pages/personalized-nutrition-quiz?srsltid=AfmBOopublIJFM-s0rQX7dKC0OdWKSCAiPAGVl HBm0es5CXy5ZZAiKTP
- Coombs, K. (Host). (2024, January 12). *#66 Taking charge of your healing journey with Dr. Krista Coombs* [Audio podcast episode]. The Positive Perimenopause Podcast. Buzzsprout. https://thepositiveperi menopausepodcast.buzzsprout.com/1950408/13401822
- Cycle Driven Life. (2023, September 15). *Promoting positive mental health: Strategies and tips.* Cycle Driven Life. https://cycledrivenlife.com/promoting-positive-mental-health-strategies-and-tips/
- D'Adamo, Peter J. (1996). *Eat right 4 your type.* G.P. Putnam's Sons.
- DiseaseFix. (n.d.). *Diet's impact on mental health: How your diet affects mental well-being.* https://www.diseasefix.com/health/the-mind-body-connection-how-your-diet-impacts-your-mental-health/
- DIY Active. (2025). *Bioma review: Digestion and weight loss probiotic review (2025 update).* https://diyactive.com/bioma-review-2024-top-probiotic-choice-for-holistic-health/
- Dorfman, J. (n.d.). *Ready...Set...Get Moving.* Julie Dorfman Nutrition. Retrieved from http://www.juliedorfman.com/blog/readysetget-moving4387024
- Dry Fasting Club. (n.d.). *IBS, SIBO, fasting, and the migrating motor complex.* Dry Fasting Club. https://www.dryfastingclub.com/podcast/ibs-sibo-fasting-and-the-migrating-motor-complex/
- Eatwell101. (n.d.). *Healthy food on a budget — 4 rules to cut your budget and keep eating balanced food.* https://www.eatwell101.com/4-rules-to-cut-your-budget-and-keep-eating-balanced-food
- EatingWell. (2023, March 15). *19 gut-healthy desserts to help you poop in the A.M.* EatingWell. Retrieved February 2, 2025, from https://www.eatingwell.com/gut-healthy-dessert-recipes-help-you-poop-8645424
- EatingWell. (2023, August 25). *7-day meal plan for a healthy gut, created by a dietitian.* EatingWell. Retrieved February 2, 2025, from https://www.

BIBLIOGRAPHY

- eatingwell.com/article/290821/7-day-meal-plan-for-a-healthy-gut-1200-calories/
- Epic Water Filters. (n.d.). *How to reduce inflammation in the body fast.* https://www.epicwaterfilters.com/blogs/quick-drips/how-to-reduce-inflammation-in-the-body-fast
- GamingEon. (n.d.). *The ultimate breakfast breakdown: Discover the healthiest morning meals to kickstart your day!* https://gamingeon.com/healthy-life/the-ultimate-breakfast-breakdown-discover-the-healthiest-morning-meals-to-kickstart-your-day/
- Gastro Girl. (n.d.). *Journey through the digestive system: Small intestine.* https://gastrogirl.com/journey-through-the-digestive-system-small-intestine/
- Goedeke, R. (n.d.). *The impact of prebiotics on gut health and autoimmune conditions.* Biosphere Nutrition. https://www.biospherenutrition.co.nz/blogs/prebiotics/the-impact-of-prebiotics-on-gut-health-and-autoimmune-conditions
- Good Foods Co-op. (n.d.). *Everything you need to know about keto: An overview.* https://goodfoods.coop/everything-you-need-to-know-about-keto-an-overview/
- Gunnars, K. (2021, June 18). *Fennel and fennel seeds: Nutrition and benefits.* Healthline. https://www.healthline.com/nutrition/fennel-and-fennel-seed-benefits
- Gunnars, K. (2021, August 31). *The 9 best teas for digestion.* Healthline. https://www.healthline.com/nutrition/tea-for-digestion
- *Gut microbiota, leaky gut, and autoimmune diseases.* (n.d.). PubMed Central. Retrieved [Month Day, Year], from https://pmc.ncbi.nlm.nih.gov/articles/PMC9271567/
- Hampton Roads Weight Loss. (n.d.). *How to overcome a weight-loss plateau.* https://hamptonroadsweightloss.com/how-to-overcome-a-weight-loss-plateau/
- Harkinson, J. (2014, March 12). *You're drinking the wrong kind of milk.* Mother Jones. https://www.motherjones.com/environment/2014/03/a1-milk-a2-milk-america/
- Harvard Health Publishing. (2018, May 16). *Fermented foods for better gut health.* Harvard Health Blog. Retrieved February 2, 2025, from https://www.health.harvard.edu/blog/fermented-foods-for-better-gut-health-2018051613841
- Harvard Health Publishing. (2018, October 1). *Mindful eating.* Harvard Health. https://www.health.harvard.edu/staying-healthy/mindful-eating

BIBLIOGRAPHY

- Harvard Health Publishing. (n.d.). The gut-brain connection. *Harvard Medical School*. Retrieved [2025], from https://www.health.harvard.edu/diseases-and-conditions/the-gut-brain-connection
- Harvard Health Publishing. (2015, November 16). *Nutritional psychiatry: Your brain on food*. Harvard Health Blog. Retrieved February 2, 2025, from https://www.health.harvard.edu/blog/nutritional-psychiatry-your-brain-on-food-201511168626
- Health.com. (2023, February 1). *Blood type diet: Guidelines, foods, benefits, risks*. Health.com. Retrieved February 2, 2025, from https://www.health.com/blood-type-diet-8663280
- Health Digest. (2024). *This is what happens to your gut when you don't get enough sleep*. HEALTH NEWS. https://giuseppezanotti.com.co/index.php/2024/01/12/this-is-what-happens-to-your-gut-when-you-dont-get-enough-sleep-health-digest/
- HealthKehr. (2023). *The vital importance of quality sleep*. https://www.healthkehr.com/2023/03/the-vital-importance-of-quality-sleep.html
- Healthline. (2023, July 19). *Natural ways to treat indigestion at home*. Healthline. Retrieved February 2, 2025, from https://www.healthline.com/health/home-remedies-for-indigestion
- Healthline. (2023, May 23). *Probiotics and prebiotics: What's the difference?* Healthline. Retrieved February 2, 2025, from https://www.healthline.com/nutrition/probiotics-and-prebiotics
- Health Monastery. (n.d.). *Turmeric uses*. https://healthmonastery.com/tag/turmeric-uses/
- Healthy Plate Gourmet. (n.d.). *Understanding micronutrients: Essential vitamins and minerals for your health*. https://www.healthyplategourmet.com/post/understanding-micronutrients-essential-vitamins-and-minerals-for-your-health
- Hebridean Tea Store. (2023, April 17). *Herbal infusions and their amazing benefits*. Hebridean Tea Store. https://hebrideanteastore.co.uk/herbal-infusions-and-their-amazing-benefits/
- Hol Health. (n.d.). *How to never be bloated again*. https://holhealth.com.au/how-to-never-be-bloated-again/
- Holistically Made. (n.d.). *Inflammation: The sneaky culprit of health issues*. https://www.holisticallymade.com/post/inflammation-the-sneaky-culprit-of-health-issues
- Huner, D. (2023, June 1). *How to use mindfulness to reach your weight loss goals*. FIT Orbit. https://www.fitorbit.com/how-to-use-mindfulness-to-reach-your-weight-loss-goals/

BIBLIOGRAPHY

- Innerbody. (n.d.). *Interactive guide to the digestive system.* Innerbody. Retrieved February 2, 2025, from https://www.innerbody.com/image/digeov.html
- Integris Health. (2023, October). *Simple lifestyle changes for better gut health.* Integris Health. https://integrishealth.org/resources/on-your-health/2023/october/simple-lifestyle-changes-for-better-gut-health
- Jones, T. (2021, October 14). *Does food combining work?* Healthline. https://www.healthline.comhttps://www.healthline.com/nutrition/food-combining
- Jones, T. (n.d.). *The art of mindful eating: Cultivating a balanced and joyful relationship with food.* Renew Counseling. https://renew-counseling.org/the-art-of-mindful-eating-cultivating-a-balanced-and-joyful-relationship-with-food/
- Kadooka, Y., Sato, M., Kawai, Y., Takano, Y., Ogawa, H., Miyoshi, M., Uenishi, H., Fujiya, H., & Yokoyama, M. (2013). Regulation of abdominal adiposity by *Lactobacillus gasseri* SBT2055 in adults with obese tendencies: A randomized controlled trial. *British Journal of Nutrition, 111*(8), 1507–1519. https://doi.org/10.1017/S0007114512004971
- Kern, P. A., Ranganathan, S., & Morell, M. (2013). ABO genotype, 'blood-type' diet and cardiometabolic risk factors: A review. *Journal of Human Nutrition and Dietetics, 26*(2), 177-182. https://doi.org/10.1111/jhn.12015
- Kobel, S. (2024, May 9). *Prebiotics for digestive wellness.* Saya Suka. https://www.sayasuka-water.com/blog-post/prebiotics-for-digestive-wellness
- Kohr, A. (2023, April 19). *How to have a more meaningful meal.* Wanderlust. https://wanderlust.com/de/journal/feed-soul-mindful-meal
- Kreedon. (n.d.). *Benefits of intermittent fasting | Fasting for fitness!.* https://www.kreedon.com/web-stories/benefits-of-intermittent-fasting/
- Kurniawan, R. (2023, October 16). *The benefits of mindful eating.* Kykurniawan. https://kykurniawan.com/the-benefits-of-mindful-eating-1
- Lee, Y., Lee, D., & Kim, H. (2021). Do probiotics mitigate GI-induced inflammation and gut barrier dysfunction in patients with chronic gastrointestinal diseases? *Journal of Clinical Gastroenterology, 55*(9), 758-769. https://doi.org/10.1097/MCG.0000000000001609
- Li, C., Li, C., Li, J., Li, J., Zhou, Q., Wang, C., Hu, J., Hu, J., Liu, C., & Liu, C. (2024). Effects of physical exercise on the microbiota in irritable bowel syndrome. *Nutrients, 16*(16), 2657. https://doi.org/10.3390/nu16162657
- Maud. (2024, March 29). *Why your gut loves fermented foods.* How Fresh Is This Guy. https://www.howfreshisthisguy.com/why-your-gut-loves-fermented-foods/

BIBLIOGRAPHY

- Mayer, E. A., & Tillisch, K. (2011). The impact of acute and chronic stress on gastrointestinal motility. *Journal of Physiology, 589*(9), 2703–2713. https://doi.org/10.1113/JP281951
- Mayo Clinic Staff. (2022, August 23). *Lactose intolerance - Diagnosis & treatment*. Mayo Clinic. https://www.mayoclinic.org/diseases-conditions/lactose-intolerance/diagnosis-treatment/drc-20374238
- Mayo Clinic. (n.d.). Probiotics and prebiotics: What you should know. Retrieved February 2, 2025, from https://www.mayoclinic.org/healthy-lifestyle/nutrition-and-healthy-eating/expert-answers/probiotics/faq-20058065
- Medical News Today. (2023, May 9). *Complementary therapies for IBS: Diet, herbs, and more*. Medical News Today. Retrieved February 2, 2025, from https://www.medicalnewstoday.com/articles/complementary-therapies-for-ibs
- Medical News Today. (n.d.). *SIBO: Symptoms, causes, treatment, and diet*. https://www.medicalnewstoday.com/articles/324475
- Morning Lazziness. (n.d.). *10 best detox morning drinks for weight loss*. https://www.morninglazziness.com/web-stories/10-best-detox-morning-drinks-for-weight-loss/
- MySoulSpace.ie. (n.d.). *Chia berry pudding*. https://mysoulspace.ie/eat/recipe-chia-berry-pudding/
- National Institute of Diabetes and Digestive and Kidney Diseases (NIDDK). (n.d.). *Digestive diseases*. U.S. Department of Health and Human Services. Retrieved February 2, 2025, from https://www.niddk.nih.gov/health-information/digestive-diseases
- National Institute of Diabetes and Digestive and Kidney Diseases (NIDDK). (n.d.). Your digestive system & how it works. Retrieved February 2, 2025, from https://www.niddk.nih.gov/health-information/digestive-diseases/digestive-system-how-it-works
- Nicholson, J. K., & Wilson, I. D. (2024). Antibiotics and the gut microbiome: Understanding the impact. *Advances in Microbiome Research, 6*(2), 45–67. https://doi.org/10.1016/j.advmicrores.2024.00009
- No author. (n.d.). *Gut microbiome diversity is associated with sleep physiology ... [Article]*. PubMed Central. https://pmc.ncbi.nlm.nih.gov/articles/PMC6779243/
- Northeast Digestive. (n.d.). *Helping your gut on a budget*. Northeast Digestive. Retrieved February 2, 2025, from https://northeastdigestive.com/blog/helping-your-gut-on-a-budget/
- NOW Foods. (n.d.). *Food-grade essential oil FAQs - Aromatherapy*. NOW

BIBLIOGRAPHY

Foods. https://www.nowfoods.com/healthy-living/articles/food-grade-essential-oil-faqs

- Nunc Drinks. (2023, October 5). *Why fermented food and drink is important to your diet*. Nunc Drinks. https://nuncliving.com/blogs/news/why-fermented-food-and-drink-is-important-to-your-diet
- Nutrioo. (n.d.). *Blog post*. https://nutrioo.io/full_blog/115
- O'Neill, C. A., & O'Connor, P. M. (2020). *Fermented foods, health, and the gut microbiome*. PMC. https://pmc.ncbi.nlm.nih.gov/articles/PMC9003261/
- Otsuka Pharmaceutical Co., Ltd. (n.d.). *Energy production and B vitamins*. Otsuka Pharmaceutical Co., Ltd. Retrieved February 2, 2025, from https://www.otsuka.co.jp/en/nutraceutical/about/nutrition/sports-nutrition/essential-nutrients/vitaminbcomplex.html
- Patel, E. (2023, September 12). *Supercharge your immune system: Unveiling the probiotic secrets*. ProbioticsEverything. https://probioticseverything.com/supercharge-your-immune-system-unveiling-the-probiotic-secrets/
- Peninsula Integrative Medicine. (2019, October 7). *What is causing your stomach pain and how to treat it naturally*. https://peninsulaintegrative.com/2019/10/07/what-is-causing-your-stomach-pain-and-how-to-treat-it-naturally/
- Performance Food Centers. (n.d.). *Gut health smoothies to improve digestion*. Performance Food Centers. Retrieved February 2, 2025, from https://www.performancefoodcenters.com/blog/all-about-gut-health-smoothies-and-why-they-work#:~:text=Aim%20to%20blend%20up%20at,mood%20as%20your%20microbiome%20flourishes
- Reiki of Austin. (2024, January 14). *Reiki and the impact on digestive health*. https://www.reikiofaustin.com/reiki-and-the-impact-on-digestive-health
- Revolt Fitness. (2022, January 23). *Just breathe*. Revolt Fitness. https://revoltfitness.net/just-breathe/
- Rosenberg, S. (2012, February 13). *Take the Wellness Week pledge for a healthier you*. SpaFinder. https://www.spafinder.com/blog/mindset/wellness-week-pledge-healthier/
- Rothschild, D., Weissbrod, O., Barkan, E., et al. (2022). Environmental factors shaping the gut microbiome in a global population. *Nature, 608*(7921), 1–12. https://doi.org/10.1038/s41586-022-04567-7
- Royal Therapy. (n.d.). *Sleeplessness hurts us*. https://royal-therapy.com/blogs/home-page-22/sleeplessness-hurts-us-copy
- Rupa Health. (n.d.). *Anti-inflammatory eating for gut health: Connecting diet and digestion*. Retrieved February 2, 2025, from https://www.rupahealth.com/post/anti-inflammatory-eating-for-gut-health-connecting-diet-and-digestion

BIBLIOGRAPHY

- Sage Nutrition. (2022, December 6). *Introducing Sage Academy*. Sage Nutrition. https://sagenutrition.org/2022/12/06/introducing-sage-academy/
- Sally Tea Cups. (n.d.). *What does ginger turmeric tea do for you?* https://sallyteacups.org/what-does-ginger-turmeric-tea-do-for-you/
- Self, R. (2023, May 23). *Lessons from a dandelion*. GardenTabs. https://gardentabs.com/lessons-from-a-dandelion/
- Sixwise. (2009, December 18). *Help for hard-to-treat fungal infections*. http://sixwise.com/Newsletters/2009/December/18/Help-for-Hard-to-Treat-Fungal-Infections.htm
- Smart Patients. (n.d.). *Irritable Bowel Syndrome community*. Smart Patients. Retrieved February 2, 2025, from https://www.smartpatients.com/communities/ibs#:~:text=The%20Irritable%20Bowel%20Syndrome%20community,medical%20science%20for%20their%20condition
- Sonnenburg, E. D., & Sonnenburg, J. L. (2022). The gut microbiome: A core regulator of metabolism. *Journal of Endocrinology, 256*(3), 1–10. https://doi.org/10.1530/JOE-22-0111
- SpaFinder. (n.d.). *Take the Wellness Week pledge for a healthier you*. https://www.spafinder.com/blog/mindset/wellness-week-pledge-healthier/
- Spirko, J. (2023, October 19). *Lacto-fermentation for preservation, flavor & health – Epi-3326*. The Survival Podcast. https://www.thesurvivalpodcast.com/salt-and-time
- Suntek Lawn Care. (n.d.). *What is: Nutrient uptake efficiency*. https://sunteklawncare.com/glossario/what-is-nutrient-uptake-efficiency/
- Supplement Links. (n.d.). *Fermented foods: Boosting gut health with natural goodness*. https://supplementlinks.com/supplement/fermented-foods
- The Art of Cooking. (n.d.). *5:2 diet*. 531 Shop. https://531shop.net/tag/5-2-diet/
- The Bed Warehouse Direct. (2024). *Sleeping your way to a healthier 2024: New year resolutions for better sleep*. The Bed Warehouse Direct Blog. https://www.thebedwarehousedirect.com/blog/sleeping-your-way-to-a-healthier-2024-new-year-resolutions-for-better-sleep/
- TheCareUp. (n.d.). *Top tips to boost your health and well-being*. https://thecareup.com/top-tips-to-boost-your-health-and-well-being/
- The Gut Health Doctor. (n.d.). *Transformation stories*. The Gut Health Doctor. Retrieved February 2, 2025, from https://www.theguthealthdoctor.com/transformation-stories
- *The gut microbiome: A core regulator of metabolism in endocrine health and disease*. (2022). *Journal of Endocrinology, 256*(3), Article JOE-22-0111. https://joe.bioscientifica.com/view/journals/joe/256/3/JOE-22-0111.xml

BIBLIOGRAPHY

- The New York Banner. (n.d.). *Gut health and weight loss.* https://thenybanner.com/index.php/weight-loss/gut-health/
- Turnbaugh, P. J., Ley, R. E., Mahowald, M. A., Magrini, V., Mardis, E. R., & Gordon, J. I. (2006). Effects of gut microbes on nutrient absorption and energy regulation. *Cell Metabolism, 14*(3), 789–799. https://doi.org/10.1016/j.cmet.2006.09.012
- Turtle Tree Seeds. (n.d.). *7 weight loss smoothies packed with seed power.* https://turtletreeseeds.com/7-weight-loss-smoothies-packed-with-seed-power/
- UCLA Health. (2023, February 1). *Resetting gut microbiome is a long-term project.* UCLA Health. Retrieved February 2, 2025, from https://www.uclahealth.org/news/article/resetting-gut-microbiome-is-a-long-term-project
- Uncover Counseling. (n.d.). *The science of stress: How it affects your body.* Uncover Counseling. https://uncovercounseling.com/blog/the-science-of-stress-effect-of-stress-in-the-body/
- University of Arizona, Campus Health. (n.d.). *Irritable bowel syndrome: Diet and stress.* https://health.arizona.edu/sites/default/files/irritable_bowel_syndrome_diet_and_stress.pdf
- Unlock Food. (n.d.). *10 tips for planning meals on a budget.* Unlock Food. Retrieved February 2, 2025, from https://www.unlockfood.ca/en/Articles/Budget/10-Tips-for-Planning-Meals-on-a-Budget.aspx
- WILLY Cafe. (n.d.). *Nurturing your gut: A holistic and natural approach to healing stomach issues.* https://willycafe.com/blogs/news/nurturing-your-gut-a-holistic-and-natural-approach-to-healing-stomach-issues
- Wittmer Rejuvenation Clinic. (n.d.). *Celiac disease evaluation (TTG-A, DGP-A, TTG-G, DGP-G) blood work lab test.* Wittmer Rejuvenation Clinic. https://wittmerrejuvenationclinic.com/product/celiac-disease-evaluation-ttg-a-dgp-a-ttg-g-dgp-g/
- Yuvaap Team. (2024, February 3). *7 benefits of fermentation process for gut health.* Yuvaap. https://www.yuvaap.com/web-stories/7-benefits-of-fermentation-process-for-gut-health/
- Zhang, X., Li, Y., & Yang, T. (2023). Gut microbiota, leaky gut, and autoimmune diseases. *Frontiers in Immunology, 14,* 9271567. https://doi.org/10.3389/fimmu.2023.9271567
- Zhao, L., & Zhang, H. (2024). Editorial: Personalized nutrition and gut microbiota. *Frontiers in Nutrition, 11,* 1375157. https://doi.org/10.3389/fnut.2024.1375157

Printed in Dunstable, United Kingdom